The Intuitive Arts
on
HEALTH

The Intuitive Arts
on
HEALTH

Arlene Tognetti and Carolyn Flynn

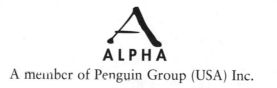

ALPHA
A member of Penguin Group (USA) Inc.

International Standard Book Number: 1-59257-109-3
Library of Congress Catalog Card Number: 2003111789

05   04   03   8   7   6   5   4   3   2   1

Interpretation of the printing code: The rightmost number of the first series of numbers is the year of the book's printing; the rightmost number of the second series of numbers is the number of the book's printing. For example, a printing code of 03-1 shows that the first printing occurred in 2003.

Printed in the United States of America

Publisher: Marie Butler-Knight
Product Manager: Phil Kitchel
Senior Managing Editor: Jennifer Chisholm
Senior Acquisitions Editor: Randy Ladenheim-Gil
Book Producer: Lee Ann Chearney/Amaranth Illuminare
Development Editor: Lynn Northrup
Copy Editor: Keith Cline
Technical Editor: Reba Jean Cain
Cover Designer: Charis Santillie
Book Designer: Trina Wurst
Creative Director: Robin Lasek
Layout/Proofreading: Angela Calvert, John Etchison

Contents

Appendixes

Introduction

Claim your brightest destiny and fulfill your own essential nature.

More than ever, we are searching for an inner awareness that brings outer confidence, joy, and direction. *The Intuitive Arts* series, with volumes on *Health, Family, Love, Money,* and *Work,* gives readers looking for answers to questions of daily living tools from the esoteric arts that will help them look deeply, see, and make real changes affecting their futures. In each problem-solving volume, curious querents are presented exercises in the Intuitive Arts of Astrology, Tarot, and Psychic Intuition that examine, instruct, illuminate, and guide. In essence, you get three books for one—but also so much more!

An understanding of the interplay of the Intuitive Arts of Astrology, Tarot, and Psychic Intuition is something most people gain slowly over time, or with the aid of a professional Intuitive Arts practitioner who already has the knowledge to give in-depth readings that link the arts together.

In *The Intuitive Arts* series, expert author Arlene Tognetti shares her deep knowing of the arts of Astrology, Tarot, and Psychic Intuition to give you the best opportunity to work out solutions to life's problems and challenges with the benefit of the sophisticated relationships between the arts Arlene reveals chapter by chapter. By combining the Intuitive Arts together throughout each chapter's exercises, you'll gain insights that link the arts together—how, for example, Tarot's Queen of Cups soothes your Psychic Intuition in an aromatherapy self-forgiveness cleansing bath. Or use Tarot's Major Arcana to deepen the energies of Astrology's power points—Sun ☉, Moon ☽, and ascendant—and intuit the strengths of your Elemental Health Signature.

Arlene Tognetti and New Age book producer Lee Ann Chearney at Amaranth Illuminare created this series for Alpha Books to respond to the public's growing fascination with all things spiritual. People (like you!) want to know how they can use the Intuitive Arts to solve everyday challenges, plan for the future, and live in the present, with hands-on advice and techniques that will make things better for them. We want to help you improve the issues surrounding *your* unique life situation by providing a multi-art approach that gives you multiple pathways to personal growth and answers your questions about health, family, love, money, and work.

Using Tarot's Major and Minor Arcana cards and spreads; Astrology's birth charts and aspect grids, sign, planets, and houses; and Psychic Intuition's meditations, affirmations, and inner knowing exercises, the innovative Intuitive Arts series provides a truly interactive, solution-oriented, positive message that enriches a personal synergy of mind, body, and spirit!

Read on to further *your* knowledge and understanding of how the Intuitive Arts work together to reveal deep insights. In this series volume, *The Intuitive Arts on Health*, learn how Astrology, the Tarot, and Psychic Intuition reveal *your* future well-being!

Are *you* ready to manifest your most vital self?

chapter 1

Live Long and Prosper!

The Intuitive Arts meet health
Your Psychic Intuition: Essence of health
Timeless wisdom: Health through the ages
Know your essence: Astrology and health
The Tarot and well-being: A walkthrough
An Intuitive Arts body scan

Health is the currency of happiness. It affects life's most essential transactions—how we love, how we work, how we know the world. Health defines who we are and how we relate to ourselves and each other. The way we view our body's strength and beauty determines the way we move through the day. At its essence, our health shapes what we believe about the divine and the eternal. So it's no wonder that no matter where you turn, the newsstands, the airwaves, cyberspace are overflowing with talk about wellness of body, mind, and spirit. We seek to live a life long, rich, and full of vitality. In this book, we show you how the Intuitive Arts can put you back into the picture of health. We believe Astrology, Tarot, and Psychic Intuition can instruct, illuminate, and guide you toward manifesting the best practices for your health. As we accompany you on this journey, we touch on some of the most ancient and enduring wisdom about health and well-being.

The Intuitive Arts Meet Health and Well-Being

In our go-go-go/achieve/acquire/do world, we measure ourselves not by who we are but what we have or accomplish. But true vitality is not about what you do; it's about *who* you are. You are meant to be your most vital self, flush with the goodness that is life. You are meant to breathe easy, to sleep peacefully, to be comfortable in your own skin, to move and experience life without physical restriction, to be the best you can be, and to fulfill your true purpose—to *feel better,* to *feel good,* to *live well.*

Your most important asset in improving health and well-being may be your own intuition about your body, your mind, and your spirit. In other words, you already possess the knowledge that can guide you on the best path to health. In this book, we use the Intuitive Arts of Astrology, Tarot, and Psychic Intuition to open you up to the healing power of your own inner knowing. We urge you to keep an Intuitive Arts notebook at hand as you experience the exercises in this book— something portable and convenient in which you can record your thoughts, ideas, and impressions.

What healing traditions through the ages share with Astrology, Tarot, and Psychic Intuition is that they, too, embrace intuitive ways of understanding our bodies, our minds, and our spirits. We show you how and where the resonances between the Intuitive Arts and the many healing traditions—from ayurveda to meditation and more—can help you learn about the health of your body, mind, and spirit, and how you can enhance it.

Timeless Wisdom

Throughout the ages, women have drawn upon maternal instinct to know how to nourish their children or nurse them when they are ill. New Mexico draws upon a long history of natural herbal healing in the *curandera,* the wise grandmotherly healer who uses natural reme- dies. Men also have held revered positions in many ancient cultures as shamans, medicine men, and physicians—for example, the Greek physi- cian Galen, who proved that blood, and not air, moves through human veins. Galen's work stood for centuries at the base of Greek, Roman, and Arabic medicine.

Discovery through intuition has always played a part in health, and it is just now, with the explosion of interest in traditional healing arts, that human intuition is being folded back into the science of conventional medicine. If nothing else, the surge of interest in natural, alternative, and integrative medicine has put the patient back into the process and resulted in scenes like this: A man in the checkout line at the natural foods grocery swears by an all-organic sugar-free cranberry concentrate for his kidney stones. He won't buy any other brand. Or, a woman uses yoga and massage to ease through premenstrual tensions.

It's clear that alternative body, mind, and spirit practices are steadily entering the mainstream—ayurveda, chiropractic, meditation, vitamin therapy, and traditional Chinese medicine techniques such as acupuncture and Chinese herbs. The National Institutes of Health now recognizes Chinese acupuncture as an accepted therapy. In 1998, the NIH established the National Center for Complementary and Alternative Medicine to identify accepted alternative medicine practices. On the global front, the World Health Organization recognizes ayurveda, a natural system of healing originating from India, as an accepted form of medicine.

Until recently, these traditional healing arts survived through oral tradition. Ayurveda is estimated to be about 5,000 years old and has influenced Chinese, Greek, Arabic, and Roman schools of medical thought—yes, including Hippocrates, the father of Western medicine. When you use aromatherapy, homeopathy, and naturopathy, you are drawing upon the ancient wisdom of ayurveda. Traditional Chinese medicine, which originated before the written word, has an oral tradition dating to before 200 to 300 B.C.E.

Western medicine has traditionally taken the approach that the body functions in a system outside that of the mind. However, ancient healing arts such as traditional Chinese medicine and ayurveda have always treated the mind and spirit as well as the physical being. Just as these ancient healing arts have survived largely through oral tradition, so have the practices of Astrology, the Tarot, and Psychic Intuition. What they share in common is they put the most important healer— you—back into the bliss center of optimal health and well-being.

Health in Popular Culture

The theme of the fountain of youth is timeless, a favorite in classic literature and popular culture, from *The Secret of Dorian Gray* by Oscar Wilde to Ron Howard's movie *Cocoon*. The allure of longevity has always tempted us, and now you can go into cyberspace and calculate it. Northwestern Life Insurance Co. offers a longevity calculator on its website (www.nmfn.com/tn/learnctr--life events--longevity). Plug in your present age, your gender, your blood pressure, your family heart history, your exercise habits, your drug and alcohol habits, your driving record, and whether you smoke—and the site will calculate your life expectancy. (However, the Intuitive Arts would advise you that *you are not a statistic!* Your life path is uniquely *your own.*)

As baby boomers age, they make aging beautiful, redefining physical beauty and leading the way to cultivating inner peace. In his early 50s, Bruce Springsteen is at the top of his art, creatively, physically, and spiritually. Oprah Winfrey, now in her late 40s, has built an entire empire from her commitment to self-improvement and self-acceptance—a talk show, a fitness regimen, a book club, and a magazine. You'll meet them and others in the pages of this book—from Goldie Hawn and daughter Kate Hudson to the Dalai Lama, Christopher Reeve, and Deepak Chopra.

In his book *Ageless Body, Timeless Mind,* Deepak Chopra caught the attention of a whole generation and ushered in a new era of body-mind-spirit health. Chopra was an endocrinologist practicing in Boston in the 1980s when he saw the importance of seeing health as a dynamic state of balance between body, mind, and spirit. Now, countless books and lectures later, he has been dubbed the poet-prophet of alternative medicine and states that his mission is "bridging the technological miracles of the West with the wisdom of the East." Other health practitioners are also leading the way—from Bernie Siegel and Andrew Weil to Christiane Northrup and medical intuitive Carolyn Myss.

Your Intuition as the Essence of Health

Look up for a minute and take in the scene around you. If you are near a window, look out. Sit comfortably, close your eyes, and breathe deep. Now, open your eyes and absorb what you see. We looked out our window, and this is what we saw:

Blue sky
Snow on the mountain
Purple finches in the Russian olive trees
A sleek black cat padding down the sidewalk
Colorful pinwheels spinning in the wind
Sunshine
Heart-shape cottonwood leaves that have fallen and turned honey-brown

A neighbor's minivan

Firewood

The city spilling from the mountain to the valley

Okay, we had a good window. But take note of what all these represent. The snow on the mountain becomes the spring runoff that becomes the river that becomes our water to drink. It is winter in Albuquerque as we write this, and the finches are among the many birds that have migrated south. This habitat provides them food and warmth through the winter months. The sunshine on the stucco wall is warming the house. The dead cottonwood leaves provide the nutrients for the soil. The minivan provides Carolyn's neighbor with transportation. The firewood provides fuel for the fireplace, which provides warmth on these crisp, cool winter nights. The city provides culture and resources for living.

We have water to drink, air to breathe, food to eat, people to love, blue sky to inspire us—and we are nourished. We are being provided for in every moment.

Take a moment to write down now all the key components about health you can think of. Here are some we thought of; add any others you can think of at the end of this list:

Nourishment	Love
Balance	Belief in the divine
Harmony	Beauty
Reverence	Belief in the eternal
Acceptance	Strength
Warmth	Stamina
Safety	Flexibility
Grace	Tolerance
Fortitude	_____
Honor	
Flow	_____
Wisdom	_____
Inner peace	_____

Already, you probably intuitively know your body's signals when you are your healthiest—and when you are not. When you get enough sleep, your cheeks are rosy and your skin is supple. You don't have dark circles under your eyes. When you are at your optimum weight, you move confidently and gracefully. When you feel good, you speak clearly. You are effective with others at your work. You are a more compassionate friend. You are more generous with your time and energy.

To get you started on the path to optimum vitality, we have developed 10 key principles that we will take to heart in this book. We use the Intuitive Arts of Astrology, Tarot, and Psychic Intuition to illuminate these as we go along.

- ☯ Know your essence
- ☯ Stay in balance
- ☯ Cultivate harmony
- ☯ Know your true purpose
- ☯ Nourish your soul
- ☯ Know your challenges
- ☯ Know how you respond to stress
- ☯ Treat yourself with reverence
- ☯ Attract wellness
- ☯ Be in the moment

Know Your Essence: Astrology and Well-Being

Let's look at how Astrology can release your natural intuition as you seek to improve your health in body, mind, and spirit. Chances are you already know your Sun ☉ sign, but a look at the Zodiac wheel of the signs can reveal more insights into your Sun sign nature, and its influence on your health and well-being.

Astro Sign	Sun ☉ Sign Dates	Keywords
Aries ♈	March 21 to April 20	Energetic, take-charge, pioneering
Taurus ♉	April 20 to May 21	Sensual, grounded, down-to-earth
Gemini ♊	May 21 to June 22	Resourceful, quick-witted, mercurial
Cancer ♋	June 22 to July 23	Empathetic, nurturing, emotional
Leo ♌	July 23 to August 22	Charismatic, fun-loving, self-confident

Astro Sign	Sun ☉ Sign Dates	Keywords
Virgo ♍	August 22 to September 22	Resourceful, practical, analyzing
Libra ♎	September 22 to October 23	Principled, balanced, harmonious
Scorpio ♏	October 23 to November 22	Passionate, powerful, profound
Sagittarius ♐	November 22 to December 22	Adventurous, fun-loving, enthusiastic
Capricorn ♑	December 22 to January 21	Serious, hard-working, responsible
Aquarius ♒	January 21 to February 19	Idealistic, humanitarian, persistent
Pisces ♓	February 19 to March 21	Spiritual, compassionate, dreamy

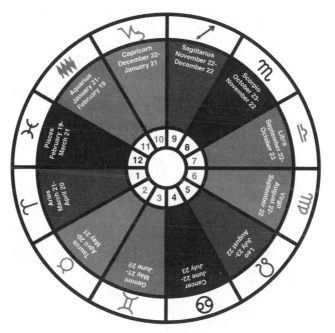

To find your Sun ☉ sign, note the name of the astrological sign that correlates to your birth date.

Parts Is Parts: A Closer Look

Each astrological sign rules certain parts of the body and can point to weak points that need to be fortified with vitamins and nutrients. Each astrological sign has natural strengths, as well as blind spots. Here's a quick glance at what the astrological signs can tell you about your body.

Astro Sign	Vitamins and Body Parts	Nutrients Needed	Health Qualities
Aries ♈	Head, face, eyes, brain	Iron; vitamin B$_{12}$	Quick thinkers; quick to anger; prone to head-aches, nervousness
Taurus ♉	Neck, throat, thyroid	Iodine; also selenium, bioflavenoids, vitamin E	Prone to slow metabolism; prone to weight gain; high endurance; solid, steady
Gemini ♊	Hands, arms, shoulders, lungs	Vitamin B complex	Great thinkers, great communicators; susceptible to headaches; sign rules connectivity
Cancer ♋	Stomach, breasts	Vitamin A; beta-carotene	Sympathetic, moody; seek comfort through food
Leo ♌	Back, spine, heart	Magnesium, calcium; pay attention to potassium and salt balance	Strength; will-power; lack of tolerance for others' weakness; prideful
Virgo ♍	Intestines, colon	Vitamin B complex; complex; PABA (para aminobenzoic acid, which maintains the health of the intestines by breaking down and using proteins)	Prone to anxiety; analyzing, dis-criminating

Astro Sign	Vitamins and Body Parts	Nutrients Needed	Health Qualities
Libra ♎	Kidneys, lower back, adrenal glands	Potassium to balance water level in kidneys; vitamin E; selenium; bioflavenoids	Harmony, balance, beauty; internalize conflict
Scorpio ♏	Genitals; urinary and reproductive system	Zinc	Great healers, with transformative powers, of selves and others; can be retentive
Sagittarius ♐	Hips, thighs, liver	Avoid excess sugar, fat, and alcohol; need vitamin K, inositol, manganese	Prone to over-indulgence; sign of locomotion; risk-taker; explorer
Capricorn ♑	Skeleton, bones, teeth	Calcium, vitamin C	Prone to arthritis, rheumatism; sign rules the process of hardening; solid, responsible
Aquarius ♒	Ankles, circulation	Magnesium	Rare illnesses; nervous ailments; forward thinking; humanitarian
Pisces ♓	Feet, immune system, hormonal system	Pantothenic acid, which stimulates the adrenal glands and boosts the immune system	Prone to addiction, overindulgence; prone to ankle sprains; compassionate; intuitive

As you look over this table, does anything resonate for you? You may already have known that your kidneys or your lower back or your intense emotions are your weak points. If you are a Libra ♎, it may have hit home with you that your kidneys need special attention. Or if you are a Pisces ♓, you may already know you have a penchant for escape in alcohol or food. Certainly it did for Carolyn, a Sagittarius Sun ♐ ☉ sign, who has always tended to overindulge in sweets (especially when she breastfed her twins!). Let's take an even closer look at how each astrological sign can influence health.

Aries ♈ March 21 to April 20. Aries, the Ram, can be impulsive and, sometimes, hotheaded. Aries are used to being pioneers, and they often are wonderful leaders because they are so inspiring to others. But they can be argumentative—sometimes they can be like steamrollers—when they want to get their way. Aries may grapple with headaches and migraines. Deep breathing helps relax Aries and sends oxygen to that busy brain!

Taurus ♉ April 20 to May 21. Taurus, the Bull, can be immovable. This stubbornness and resistance to change means Taureans are often not adaptable. The Bull has a slow metabolism and may struggle with keeping the pounds off. Emotionally, the Bull resonates to preserving the status quo instead of embracing change. On the flip side, their steadiness can mean they are the calm in the center of the storm.

Gemini ♊ May 21 to June 22. If you are a Gemini, you may wear yourself out emotionally or become mentally exhausted. Though Geminis are normally quick, clever, and adaptable, they can easily get their spirits down. If facing a long-term illness, they can often get depressed and feel hopeless—like nothing matters. These types need supporters around them to keep their spirits up. Of all the signs, Geminis probably benefit the most from meditation and calming Psychic Intuition exercises.

Cancer ♋ June 22 to July 23. Moody, sensitive Cancer isn't experiencing the world like the rest of us. Cancers dwell in the realm of emotions; and while that can make them the best when it comes to needing a sympathetic ear, it can be hard to be the one absorbing all the emotions. Cancer's tendency is to be too self-sacrificing. Cancer can be touchy—both literally and figuratively! And Cancer also feels the strong polar opposites of hot and cold more keenly than the rest of us do.

Leo ♌ July 23 to August 22. Exuberance, courage, and strength define Leo. Leo the Lion may exude health, and it may be contagious. Because Leo rules the spine, the back, and the heart—the core of the body—they rarely have physical problems. Leos are strong. But they are not as strong emotionally and do not tend to their emotions as much as others. They expect and demand adoration, because that's what feeds them, and when they don't get the worship they feel they deserve, they can become physically ill. It's important for Leos to address the under-lying emotions that contribute to physical ailments. When a Leo feels out of balance, a chiropractic adjustment or dealing with possible blood pressure problems may help restore well-being.

Virgo ♍ August 22 to September 22. A Virgo's natural fascination with both the sacred and mundane workings of all things in heaven and on earth leads them to an avid knowledge of health information. Virgos make a point to learn about the most effective vitamins or herbal remedies. Virgos, however, may tend to serve everyone else so much they don't tend to themselves. Virgos like to work, so sometimes they can be workaholics. These are people who need remedial training on relaxation, because it doesn't come naturally. All that analyzing can lead to anxiety.

Libra ♎ September 22 to October 23. Libra is always seeking equi-librium. Libra values harmony and beauty above all. But the Libran tendency to avoid discord often means they keep too much inside. They need to be prompted to pay attention to inner fitness as well as outer. Libra's Scales may find their balancing act brings strain to the adrenal glands or even lower back pain. Drink plenty of fluids to keep your kidneys in balance and practice stress-reduction techniques such as meditation, aromatherapy baths, and relaxing yoga stretches.

Scorpio ♏ October 23 to November 22. Scorpio is about getting to the root of things. They are intense, powerful, and sometimes possessive. Scorpio rules the genitals and reproductive system—and Scorpions' sexuality is potent. Those born under Scorpio have the potential to be great healers and have transformative powers, but their biggest challenge is in relinquishing negative emotions that may even-tually manifest as physical problems that have the characteristic of "holding things in" such as constipation. Scorpions should pay a lot of attention to what they eat and drink because their intake greatly influences how they think and feel.

Sagittarius ♐ November 22 to December 22. As the Archer, Sagit-tarius thrives on seeking life's basic truths. They require independence and freedom, and change does not scare them off—it enthralls them. They are optimistic—often blindly so—and that can come in handy when it comes to mind-over-matter healing. A Sagittarian is more likely to be adventurous about health—to take a "why not" approach to try-ing new approaches to healing. A Sagittarian weakness is forgetting to slow down. They can easily get overcommitted and run themselves to exhaustion.

Capricorn ♑ **December 22 to January 21.** Longevity is one of the blessings of being a Capricorn. Maybe it's all that patience. But pessimism is part of the health picture, too, and that can make a Capricorn susceptible to melancholy. Capricorns thrive in seeking out modalities that increase movement and range of motion, as Capricorn rules the bones, teeth, and skeletal structure of the body. Calcium citrate supplements can be especially helpful.

Aquarius ≈ January 21 to February 19. Independent, free-thinking Aquarians are so concerned about humanity they may neglect their own well-being! The Water Bearer can become isolated from the physical body and float in the realm of airy intellectualism and spiritual detachment. Aquarian emotions tend to come out when they are fighting for a cause or guiding a group to discover new territory. To keep circulation moving and promote body awareness, Aquarians would do well with low-impact aerobics that get the heart pumping with oxygen flowing in and also strengthen the legs and ankles.

Pisces ♓ February 19 to March 21. The challenges for intuitive, dreamy Pisces are in boundaries and addictions. Because Pisces are so sensitive to the vibrations of others, they may lose sight sometimes of where their feelings end and others' feelings begin. Pisces react poorly to environmental toxins and need to drink plenty of water to keep their bodies flushed and immune systems functioning optimally. Pisces respond best to health practices that nurture body, mind, and spirit—especially foot reflexology, as Pisces rules the feet!

Your Astrological Birth Chart: Beyond Sun ☉ Signs

You've had a glimpse of your Sun ☉ sign and your health and well-being. In exploring the Intuitive Art of Astrology throughout this book, we take you far beyond your Sun sign, to look deeply into your astrological birth chart. Your birth chart shows the heavens at the exact place and time you were born. As such, it is a map of the heavens that is uniquely *you*. When Arlene wants to know someone, she does a birth chart with the Sun ☉, the Moon ☽, the ascendant (or rising sign), and all the planets in the astrological houses.

The planets all have their own meaning and influence in Astrology. Here's a quick reference guide to each planet, with keywords to help you remember their individual healing powers as you explore your own astrological birth chart.

Astro Planet	**Keywords**
Sun ☉	Self, will, creativity
Moon ☽	Emotions, unconscious
Mercury ☿	Intelligence, communication
Venus ♀	Love, resources, harmony
Mars ♂	Ego, energy, desires
Jupiter ♃	Wisdom, growth, education
Saturn ♄	Discipline, responsibility
Uranus ♅	Intuition, originality
Neptune ♆	Spirituality, idealism
Pluto ♇	Transformation, power

Notice on your astrological birth chart that there are 12 segments on the wheel of the Zodiac; these are the astrological houses. The 1st house appears just below the eastern horizon on your chart, and the sign on its cusp is your ascendant, or your rising sign. The other houses follow counterclockwise around your birth chart. Each house represents an arena of life—12 life projects. In these houses, the lessons of your life unfold. How you learn those lessons can profoundly influence your health and well-being.

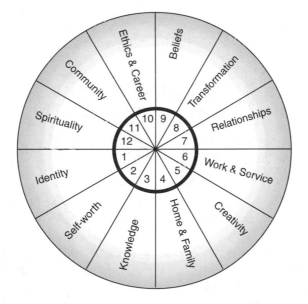

Each astrological house represents an area of your life.

To get you familiar with interpreting a birth chart, let's take a look at the Sun ☉, the Moon ☽, and the ascendant in the birth chart of poet Maya Angelou, someone who definitely represents health and longevity.

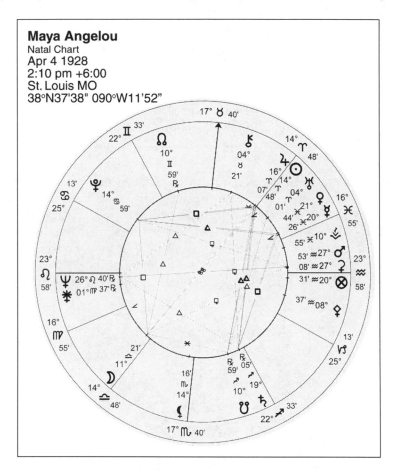

Maya Angelou
Natal Chart
Apr 4 1928
2:10 pm +6:00
St. Louis MO
38°N37'38" 090°W11'52"

Maya Angelou's birth chart.

Maya Angelou's Sun ☉ sign is in Aries ♈ in the 8th house of transformation, rebirth, and joint resources. Your Sun sign—the one most people are familiar with in casual conversation—is about your sense of self, your vitality, and your purpose. It is the strongest representation of who you are. Maya's Sun ☉ placement indicates that she is moving full speed ahead in her lifelong quest to grow and evolve personally— and to share what she has learned with us. Maya Angelou's Moon ☽ is

14

in Libra ♎ in the 2nd house of self-worth and earning potential. Your Moon sign is the inner you, your emotions, your instincts, your intuition. The Moon sign rules the subconscious, your past memories, and the dream world. Where it plays into your health is in understanding how you experience your emotions. Maya's Moon ☽ placement shows her need to balance her drive for emotional growth with the practical concerns of earning a living. In Maya Angelou's birth chart, Leo ♌ rises over the eastern horizon as her ascendant. The ascendant (or rising sign) in your birth chart tells you two key aspects of yourself. One, the ascendant represents how others perceive you. Two, it points to the skills you are learning to develop over a lifetime. With a Leo ascendant, Maya projects a bold and large-hearted persona and she's done a magnificent job in nurturing these qualities in herself.

Now, it is your turn to identify Maya's other planets, signs, and houses by completing the following table. We've gotten you started.

Maya Angelou's Planets in Their Signs and Houses

Planet	Planet Keyword	Astro Sign and Symbol	Astro Sign Keyword	House	House Keyword
Sun ☉	Self	Aries ♈	Energetic	8th	Transformation
Moon ☽	Emotion	Libra ♎	Harmony	2nd	Self-worth
Mercury ☿	_____	_____	_____	_____	_____
Venus ♀	_____	_____	_____	_____	_____
Mars ♂	_____	_____	_____	_____	_____
Jupiter ♃	_____	_____	_____	_____	_____
Saturn ♄	_____	_____	_____	_____	_____
Uranus ♅	_____	_____	_____	_____	_____
Neptune ♆	_____	_____	_____	_____	_____
Pluto ♇	_____	_____	_____	_____	_____

To generate your own astrological birth chart, you need to know the day, year, and time of your birth, as well as the place of your birth. If you don't know your precise birth time, try to narrow it down to morning, afternoon, or evening. If it is impossible to determine anything more than the day and year of birth, then use noon as your birth time.

Arlene used the computer software program Solar Fire 5, published by Astrolabe, Inc., to generate the birth charts we've adapted as examples throughout this book. Charts are cast using the Geocentric View, Tropical Zodiac, Placidus House system, and True Node because these are the most common in modern Western Astrology. To use your birth chart with this book, you need to be sure to specify these parameters when generating your own astrological birth chart. You can order a birth chart online or from your local metaphysical bookstore; there's more information on how to order a birth chart in Appendix A at the back of this book.

It is possible to learn much about yourself, your health, and your well-being from this book without having your birth chart in hand. However, we highly recommend that you take the time to generate and explore your astrological birth chart. Begin by creating a table in your Intuitive Arts notebook of the planets and signs in their houses as revealed in *your* astrological birth chart, as we've done for Maya Angelou. Soon the signs and symbols will be second nature.

Bon Voyage: Tarot's High Priestess

We continue our intuition journey with an introduction to the Tarot through one of its symbolic figures: the High Priestess card from the Major Arcana.

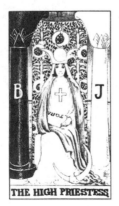

Tarot's High Priestess is the gatekeeper of intuition.

The High Priestess represents our subconscious knowledge and intuitive awareness—new ways of taking in information. Have you ever heard the phrase "listening to your gut"? Well, that's the High

Priestess. Take a moment to study this woman, with a crescent moon at her feet and the full and crescent moons on her crown. Just like Astrology's Moon ☽, she represents seeing the world in a new kind of light.

What the Tarot Tells You About Your Health

Think of the Tarot as telling you a story about yourself. Just as dreams can unlock clues from your subconscious, so can the Tarot. Tarot is as ancient as the stuff of dreams, dating back as many as 15,000 years. It has roots in China, the Middle East, and Egyptian hieroglyphics, as well as in the Hebrew Kabbalah. Tarot was often seen as a way of talking to God, of seeking to know divine will.

Each of the 78 Tarot cards depicts a scene. Because the imagery of a Tarot deck often includes universal symbols—such as a crown or a star—or biblical, mythical, or archetypal figures, they can be easy and fun to interpret. The Tarot represents the mysteries of the ages, the stories and myths we have collected over time to illuminate our worlds with meaning. They represent a pictorial convergence of many cultures and traditions in an attempt to explain events that surpass modern science's ability to explain.

The journey of life represented in Tarot's 22 Major Arcana cards starts with the Fool, who represents innocence and beginnings, and ends with the World, the card of self-actualization and attainment. Each Major Arcana card depicts steps on the journey to enlightenment, with each representing a fork in the road where you must make a choice.

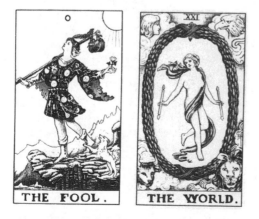

The journey of well-being starts with the Fool's innocence and completes with the World.

A quick tour through Tarot's Major Arcana yields these symbols: Our friend the High Priestess represents the Jungian archetype of *anima,* the female spirit, while the Sun might represent the Divine Child. The three archangels—Michael, Raphael, and Gabriel—appear in various cards. The Lovers card evokes Adam and Eve, while the Devil picks up in the Garden of Eden at the moment of temptation. The Wheel of Fortune card depicts a sphinx (as does the Chariot), as well as four astrological signs. The knight on the Death card reminds us of the time of King Arthur.

Take a moment to go through your Tarot deck, separate out the Major Arcana cards, and get acquainted with their imagery. Make some notes about what the images evoke for you. We have given you some categories as prompts, but this is just a beginning:

Symbol or Archetype	Tarot Card Evoked and Intuitive Notes
Mythical	
Apollo, Greek god of the sun	_____
Aphrodite, Greek goddess of love	_____
Diana, Roman goddess of the Moon, fertility, and the hunt	_____
Pomegranate (myth of Persephone)	_____
Biblical	
Prodigal son	_____
Archangels	_____
Garden of Eden	_____
Judgment day	_____
Tower of Babel	_____
Archetypal	
Wise old man	_____
The trickster	_____
The persona	_____
The darkness	_____

Symbol or Archetype	Tarot Card Evoked and Intuitive Notes
Animus	_____
Anima	_____
The Great Mother	_____
Ancient cultures/historical figures	
Sphinx	_____
King Arthur	_____
Astrological signs	
Libra ♎ (fairness and justice)	_____
Aquarius ♒ (intellectual innovation)	_____
Scorpio ♏ (passion)	_____
Taurus ♉ (stability)	_____
Leo ♌ (lion-hearted)	_____

Did you find the pomegranates in the High Priestess—and did you remember the role pomegranate seeds played in the myth of Persephone, which bears the themes of fecundity and the Great Mother? And did you see the Aquarian ♒ Water-Bearer in the Moon card? The prodigal son in the Fool?

The 56 Minor Arcana cards are broken down into suits—just like a deck of playing cards full of hearts, clubs, diamonds, and spades, except there are no trump cards here! In Tarot, the suits are Wands, Pentacles, Cups, and Swords, and they do have a King, Queen, Knight, and Page. The Minor Arcana represent the choices we make in our everyday lives. These are often referred to as the free-will cards, while the Major Arcana are the destiny cards. Another way of putting it is that the Major Arcana reflect your karma—your particular spiritual path and the lessons you need to learn in life—while the Minor Arcana inform you about your day-to-day choices.

Most of the Tarot's Minor Arcana have very affirming, positive messages about your health. Some Minor Arcana cards, though, specifically relate to certain conditions. Stress is revealed when the 5 of Wands and the 10 of Wands come up. Emotional pain is represented in the 5 of

Cups and the 8 of Cups. It's easy to guess that the suit of Swords often depicts pain—ouch!—but it can also signify loss of stamina and courage. The 3 of Swords can indicate pain and depression. The 9 of Swords can indicate depression. Because Pentacles are associated with coins—or money—the presence of Pentacles often can be interpreted as impoverishment of the body, soul, or Earth. Too many Pentacles in a Tarot reading about a question of health could point to poor nutrition or not enough sleep.

In interpreting a Tarot reading, three factors are considered—the meaning of the card, its position, and its timing. Often the position determines whether an issue that comes up in Tarot is one that has shaped your past, is in your present, or will influence your future. In some of the more complex spreads, however, such as the Horoscope Spread you'll do in Chapter 9, position can have more intricate connotations. A reversed, or upside-down, card in a reading might indicate that the positive energy of the card is blocked and requires release. A reversed card can point you directly to the area where some health work needs to be done. Tarot cards also reveal time frames as part of their meaning.

Tarot Cards	Tarot Timing
Ace through 10	1 to 10 days, weeks, or months (depending on the card)
Page	11 days, weeks, or months
Knight	12 days, weeks, or months
Queen and King	Unknown time—it's up to you!

Tarot Suits	Tarot Suit Timing
Wands	Days to weeks/spring
Cups	Weeks to months/summer
Swords	Days, fast!/fall
Pentacles	Months to years/winter

The numbers on the Tarot cards also have symbolic meaning. The Minor Arcana cards, after the royal cards, are number Ace (or 1) through 10. The Major Arcana cards are numbered 1 through 22. Their base number can be determined by adding the numbers together. For example, for Temperance, card 14, add 1 and 4 to receive the sum of 5; it makes sense that Temperance would resonate to the number of change, which definitely requires patience!

Number	Symbolic Meaning
1	Drive and determination
2	Balance and union
3	Creative enthusiasm
4	Practical planning
5	Impulsive spontaneity
6	Nurturing concern
7	Serene contemplation
8	Powerful achievement
9	Spiritual completion

For this book, we are using the Universal Waite Tarot Deck published by U.S. Games Systems, Inc. However, you should feel free to explore the many Tarot decks available and use a deck that resonates to you intuitively.

The Tarot and Health: A Walkthrough

Starting with the 22 Major Arcana cards, go through each card one by one. Which cards seem to speak to you particularly about health? Make notes in your Intuitive Arts notebook about what you feel their messages are. Our walkthrough yielded five cards: the Empress, the Chariot, the Hermit, the Star, and Judgement.

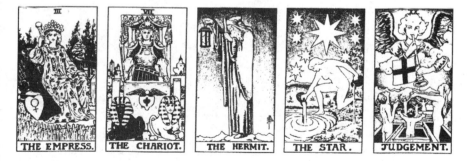

These Major Arcana cards speak to us with archetypal messages about well-being.

Why? **The Empress** is about abundance and fertility—the archetypal Earth Mother. She represents comfort and an emotionally supportive environment. When **the Chariot** comes up, it's about success in overcoming illness or adversity. The Chariot represents stamina. **The Hermit** is the archetypal sage or medicine man. When the Hermit card comes up, it's a signal to seek wise advice about your health. It's a time to get introspective, to reflect on the advice from medical professionals and listen to your inner wisdom. **The Star** card is that of hope and faith. It tells you that you can heal anything. It's the card of optimism. **Judgement** is the card of awakening. It signals that better health is to come, that you will see what you need to do about your health. It signals that you will be strong in your convictions to recuperate and to create a better chance at health and longevity. Ahead lies a better quality of life.

Take a moment to pick five more cards at random from your Tarot deck, and you need not limit yourself to the Major Arcana; consider the Minor Arcana cards as well. For each card, answer these questions:

- ☯ What is this card telling you about your health?
- ☯ What do you feel you already know about your health?

Now, choose three keywords for each card and note them in your Intuitive Arts notebook. Before we go into the next chapters and start doing Tarot spreads and readings, you'll want to take some time to familiarize yourself with the rest of your deck. In Appendix B, we have provided pictures of all cards in the Universal Waite Tarot Deck, along with keywords highlighting their messages about health. This can be a handy reference for you as you get acquainted with the cards.

Reactivating Your Psychic Intuition

A popular bumper sticker says, "Reality is the leading cause of stress." Cancer and AIDS may dominate the health research being done in the world's leading medical labs, but the most common disease for all of us is chronic stress. A host of other diseases—some scientifically documented, others we only know through deep intuition—stem from this one source. Of course, there's good stress and bad stress; but whether it's good (new job, new baby) or bad (layoff, divorce), it's stress, stress, stress. Stress is a part of life; it's how we respond to stress that makes the difference.

Physician, researcher, and founder of the Mind/Body Medical Institute Herbert Benson discovered the physiological changes that occur during deep meditation: reduced heart rate, blood pressure, and oxygen consumption; release of muscular tension; raised skin temperature and altered brain-wave patterns. These positive physiological effects of a calm mental state were termed the "relaxation response," and Benson believed it to be inborn. That is, we all have the ability to do it. It's built into the human design.

The combination of breath awareness and body-scan relaxation can bring you back into awareness of energy that is blocked in your body, holding you back from your best opportunity for health. When we become anxious, we tend to hold our breath. Over time, this becomes a habit, and we become shallow breathers, just barely filling our lungs with each breath. This keeps our bodies in a perpetual state of alarm, as if we are in a constant "flight or fight" response. Arlene is quick to acknowledge that this is one of her weak areas. "I have to remember to breathe deep; if I don't, only more anxiety comes in" is the way she puts it. Breath focus can break the vicious cycle. In breath focus, we breathe in, allowing the breath to reach into all the tense and negative areas in our bodies with its healing calm. Then, we hold the breath in a cleansing pause. Finally, we exhale the breath fully and deeply as we smile with the release of positive, rejuvenating energy.

A body scan reveals to you more than just the areas that are blocked: It trains your mind to get more connected with your body. Remember that our bodies are informing us constantly of what they need and how they work. It is we who have shut ourselves off from this constant flow of information. Our bodies carry tension in different parts; some of those parts may have been aching for years. Know also that our bodies hold a memory map of all of our physical and emotional injuries. A body scan begins with deep breathing and breath focus, and works its way through the seven chakras, or energy centers (more about the chakras in Chapter 6). As you do a body scan, you will discover tensions you didn't know were stored up in your body. Feelings that you didn't know you had stored up will be released. Once you hone the practice of body scanning, you will be more effective at it. You may be able to release strain on a muscle by returning to a simple awareness of your breathing moving into that muscle and pushing out the tension.

Simple meditation practice, such as the body scan that follows, is the best way to cultivate your Psychic Intuition. Psychic Intuition is simply listening to your inner center of bliss. If you have ever had a hunch or an insight or "just a feeling" about a person, place, or thing that turned out to resonate with truth, you have experienced Psychic Intuition.

Body Scan

First, get in a comfortable place. Most people find lying down is the best way to do this. Make sure you are not too warm or too cold, because that will distract you. Then, close your eyes, and let all thoughts fall away as you take in deep breaths. After your mind is blank, begin to pay attention to your breathing. Allow your stomach to rise as you inhale and fall as you exhale. Concentrate on your forehead first. Become aware of any muscle tension there. As you breathe out, release the tension in those muscles. Imagine sending your breath out through your forehead, loosening and softening those muscles, gently pushing them away.

Now repeat the process, working through these areas: eyes and the muscles around them; mouth and jaw; throat and neck; back; shoulders; upper arms; lower arms; chest; stomach; pelvis and buttocks; upper legs; and lower legs, ankles, and feet. If you lose your concentration, move your thoughts back to your stomach as it rises with each exhalation.

As you do this, do any parts take longer to relax? Do any of them surprise you?

The Journey Ahead

Once you re-activate your body, mind, and spirit awareness through the Intuitive Arts of Astrology, Tarot, and Psychic Intuition, you can set yourself on the path for lifelong vitality. In the following two chapters, we delve a little further into Astrology, Tarot, and Psychic Intuition through the use of *yin/yang* and the four Elements. Then we guide you through ways to attract your best possible health, as well as through the rocky times when the health that you once took for granted seems elusive.

chapter 2

Yin and Yang: The Balance of Feeling Good

Yin and *yang* meditation
The essence of opposites in health
The best of *yin*, the best of *yang*
Who are you in mind, body, and spirit? *Yin* and *yang* meet Astrology
Moon time: When to *yin* and when to *yang*
Yin and *yang* meet Tarot
The science of opposites: *Yin/yang* and ayurveda

Yin and yang has its origin in traditional Chinese medicine. It is the symbol for the unity of opposites, and understanding this duality in balance is the foundation of lifelong vitality. The two opposing yet complementary forces of life are in everything. All organs; all energy forces; all muscles; all tissues; all thoughts, feelings, and emotions are housed in a system of opposing yet mutually dependent forces—a constantly flowing, changing system that is you. In this chapter, we use the Intuitive Arts of Astrology, Tarot, and Psychic Intuition to understand how balancing yin *and* yang *can lead to the healthiest, happiest you.*

What Are Yin and Yang?

The symbol of *yin* and *yang* has had enduring power through the centuries because of its simplicity—yet it is very complex. It is a dynamic image, always changing, for *yin* becomes *yang* becomes *yin* again. Each opposite contains the seed of the other.

To show you what we mean: Winter solstice is the darkest day of the year, yet it has been celebrated by the ancients through the ages. Because of the winter solstice festivals, the Christian church chose to celebrate December 25 as Christ's birthday. The Christians knew a good thing when they saw it! That's because from winter solstice forward, the ancients believed, humanity heads toward the light. The ancients celebrated the return of light amid the darkest dark of the longest night of the year. Think about it. We would not have an understanding of light if not for darkness, of joy if not for sadness. The old saying is, "It's always darkest just before the dawn."

Many believe that the earliest origin of the *yin/yang* symbol came from the observation of day turning to night and night turning to day. That's right—from watching the Sun, the Moon, the planets, and the stars. The ancient Chinese charted out the days of the calendar in a circle, dividing it evenly into 24 segments and then recording the length of the shadow of the Sun each day. Connecting each line resulted in the *yin/yang* curve. Marking a dot on winter solstice and summer solstice resulted in the "eye" of *yin/yang*—the seed of the other. The first day of *yang* is winter solstice.

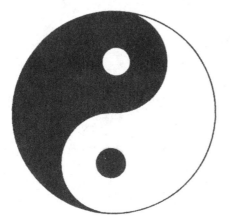

Yin *and* yang *mark the balance of summer and winter solstice and the turning of the year.*

Most of us are most familiar with *yin/yang* as the concept of complementary feminine and masculine qualities. It's the easiest way to understand it, because we are culturally attuned to define certain qualities as masculine or feminine. Check in 100 years from now, as our cultural messages about masculinity and femininity change—when it's no longer a media phenomenon if a father changes a diaper nor is it sitcom material when a ballsy female in a tight skirt mixes it up with corporate executives—and it might be a different story. But *yin/yang* goes beyond masculine/feminine. Let's take a closer look.

Yin/yang breaks down into five key concepts:

Key Concept	Definition	Example
Opposition	Two forces are in constant struggle.	Ocean/beach
Mutual dependence	One cannot exist without the other.	Male/female Up/down In/out
Mutual consumption and support	Each gives of itself to support the other.	Cow/pasture
Inter-transformation	One becomes the other.	Night/day
Infinite sub-divisibility	There is always a bit of one in the other.	Joy/sadness

Let's take a moment to brainstorm some *yin/yang* pairs. Here are some that Arlene and Carolyn collected. We have left some room for your own. Try to add in five, one for each key concept.

Yin	Yang
Earth	Heaven
Night	Day
Dark	Light
Female	Male
Moon	Sun
Autumn, winter	Spring, summer
Rest	Creation
Cold, coolness	Heat, warmth
Stillness	Movement
Inside, interior	Outside, surface
Things small, weak	Things big, powerful
The lower part	The upper part
Water, rain	Fire, Earth
The right side	The left side
West, north	East, south
Cloud	Rain

Yin	Yang
Falling	Rising
Contracting	Expanding
Soft	Hard
Intuition	Cognition
Conservation	Destruction
Responsiveness	Aggressiveness
Nurturing	Growing
Circle	Staff
Feel, sense	Act

_____   _____

_____   _____

One of our favorite pairs is cloud/rain because it has the simplicity of haiku. It is a dynamic definition. One becomes the other becoming the other again. One is a vessel for the other. Rain could not exist without a cloud. When the cloud releases the rain, the cloud ceases to exist. But the rain fills the meandering riverbeds and vast oceans that evaporate and become the cloud again.

Yin and Yang Meditation

Take a moment to meditate on the *yin/yang* symbol. You may want to sit on the floor with pillows around you. Or perhaps you may want to sit in the light of the Sun flowing through your window, warming your face. The main thing is to be comfortable in a quiet room. Take a few deep breaths. Clear your mind. As thoughts arise, don't grasp them or dwell on them—but also don't try to suppress them. Let each thought pass in peace. In just a few minutes—you will be surprised how quickly—your mind settles into calm. Release any thoughts of where you were earlier. Work gone ... traffic gone ... anxiety about next Monday gone ... only peaceful contemplative self exists now.

Imagine the *yin/yang* symbol floating in front of you. As each part flows into the other, it creates a circle of perfect wholeness. Sit for a moment in your own perfect wholeness, seeing in your mind's eye your own body in its wholeness. Sit in the flow of the doing and the undoing, the creating and waiting, the expanding and contracting of your lungs, the pumping of blood (*yang*) and the receiving of the blood (*yin*). Know that all is working as it should be. See in this flow the two forces that are in constant opposition to one another, endlessly reshaping the other. Hold yourself there in that paradox, that two forces can be in constant struggle, yet require each other to be in balance in order to exist. Hold yourself there in that harmony until you no longer are seeing but just feeling. When Carolyn did this meditation, it came to her in vivid, moving color. The *yang* part of the circle was a sunset orange, a cascade of fire flowing into the *yin* of calm blue, a sparkling, rippling wave of water.

The Essence of Opposites in Health

Yin/yang forms the foundation of traditional Chinese medicine, as do opposites in the system of ayurvedic medicine, which originated in India. But did you know that the concept of polarities works in conventional medicine as well? Vaccination is one example. To keep us from getting chicken pox, we are exposed to a little bit of the chicken pox virus. Our body's natural immune-fighting properties kick in to oppose the exposure to the virus, and—*voilà!*—no more chicken pox. Allergy shots work the same way by exposing the patient to a small amount of the irritant, building up resistance over time. The opposite can heal you.

Understand that disease and health exist in this same *yin/yang* dynamic. Whether it's a common cold or cancer, the potential for disease and health co-exist within your body. In the case of the common cold, many of us blast our bodies with symptom-relief medication, but the reality is, modern science has not developed a cure for the common cold, and so the cold virus sticks around for roughly seven days, then moves on out. Your immune system and the cold virus engage in a tension of push and pull. For seven days, this nasty virus and you are one.

In the Western world, we often talk in aggressive terms about our health. We "fight a cold" or "battle allergies." The cold virus and allergens are all part of the *yin/yang* dynamic of your body. One friend of Carolyn's who suffered from allergies recently shifted her perception of her own personal springtime irritant. Rather than treat the pollen that gives her fits as a foreigner—an alien to make battle with—the friend began to visualize encompassing the allergen in all that defined her. She visualized embracing her enemy, sending love and compassion to it. Her efforts defused all the energy she had built up around fighting the allergies. This friend accepted the pollen as part of her and who she is. "I don't like you but I'm going to have to live with you." Now, her allergies are not as intense (or as intensely experienced).

In what areas do you feel at battle with your body? Do you plow ahead when you get a nasty cold and never rest—then come down with bronchitis? Do you burn the candle at both ends? Do you fight with fluctuating weight? Are you kind and encouraging with yourself? Or do you send health messages to yourself in ways that if you made the same remarks to another person, that person would call you emotionally abusive? Do you let emotional upsets send you into depression, leave you susceptible to a cold, or diminish your effectiveness at work? Do you let toxic emotions such as anger store up inside? Take a few moments to reflect on ways you might create your own disharmony within your body. You may use the space here or write in your Intuitive Arts notebook.

_____

_____

_____

Understanding *yin/yang* is about balance. It's about promoting harmony within, even when disease or toxic thoughts or low self-esteem are part of the picture. You're not supposed to *not* have any of these things. We all have and do at one point or another. The presence of any of these is the signal that *yin/yang* is out of balance and needs to be restored.

The Best of Yin, the Best of Yang

As long as *yin* and *yang* maintain their dynamic oscillating balance, life exists. When the extremes of life's cycles oscillate closer to the center, less illness occurs, and we have optimum vitality. It is when *yin* and *yang* are out of balance that we get ill. Traditional Chinese medicine believes that if *yin* and *yang* separate, the life ceases to exist. In the body, *yin* refers to the more passive processes. Think of water. *Yin* rules the fluid and the tissue, the infrastructure and support system. Think: Blood, the lymph system, the hormonal system, your flesh, your bones. *Yang,* on the other hand, comprises the direct and active processes. *Yang* is the fire, the driving spark, of the body. *Yang* refers to our energy, our mental activity, and our spiritual process.

If you think of *yin* as the fluid of the body, then it only makes sense to describe the common cold as *yin* that is out of balance. When you are suffering from a cold, your body is overflowing with mucus deposits. Your sinuses, your throat, your lungs are clogged with too much *yin*. That's why hot foods seem to help. In New Mexico, where Carolyn lives, the first thing people do when a cold is coming on is go out and get some green chile. Not vitamin C, not grapefruit extract, not echinacea with goldenseal—but green chile, the state food. Many believe green chile stimulates the endorphins that kick into action against the cold virus. In ayurveda, ginger might be the substance of choice. Ginger's qualities are hot, ascending, and dispersing—all *yang* qualities. Those qualities help dry up the *yin* and drive out the invader.

In Chinese medicine, *yin* and *yang* each relate to certain organs and to the body's meridians, or energy points. All of the *yin* organs are solid; the *yang* organs are hollow.

Each of these *yin/yang* pairs are connected with greater and lesser energy meridians.

Yin	Yang
Lungs	Large intestine
Spleen	Stomach
Heart	Small intestine
Kidneys	Urinary tract, bladder
Pericardium (sac surrounding the heart)	Triple burner (an organ function)
Liver	Gallbladder

Who Are You in Mind, Body, and Spirit?

Each of the 12 astrological signs is defined by an energy—either *yin* or *yang*. This energy, along with the Elements (coming up in Chapter 3) and the qualities (coming up in Chapter 5), defines each astrological sign.

Yin	Yang
Taurus ♉	Aries ♈
Cancer ♋	Gemini ♊
Virgo ♍	Leo ♌
Scorpio ♏	Libra ♎
Capricorn ♑	Sagittarius ♐
Pisces ♓	Aquarius ♒

Yang signs tend to take direct action on their health. They are the type who are on the Internet all night after hearing a diagnosis from a doctor. They are the type who ask a lot of questions, and they want to be doing something about it—getting on a treadmill or eliminating salt and fat from their diets. They are uncomfortable with waiting or monitoring—they want the doctor to do something! The flip side of this is they have a hard time with acceptance and may go through a longer, stronger denial.

Yin signs are those who may take the approach of attracting the positive health they need, like a flower that blooms in order to attract a honeybee. They may take a more internal approach, tuning in to their bodies, listening to their bodies more intuitively and effecting internal changes.

Both approaches are vital to balancing your health. There is a time for proactively working on your body and restoring your health, cultivating the habits that promote your best health and seeking the information and resources that will keep you on track for healing. And there is a time for patience, watching, and inner knowing. There is a time for cultivating the peace within that will restore you for the next round if you are facing a chronic or serious health problem. That inner peace may boost your immunity or your endorphins, and the *yin* path may be the path to healing.

Certain Tarot cards can signal to you whether it's time to *yin*—or time to *yang*. The 4 of Wands may signal to you that it's time to gather family and friends around you and celebrate a joyful time. It may come up after a period of doing a lot of hard work on your health, whether you have overcome depression, lost a ton of weight, survived a nasty divorce, or your illness is in remission. When this card comes up, it's time to rest and celebrate the moment of being alive. Know that you have done all you can do for now, and you have done well. It was time to *yang* when Carolyn was in the last trimester of her pregnancy with the twins, having preterm labor and facing a possible Cesarean. The Queen of Swords came up for Carolyn, telling her to fight for those children with fierceness and courage.

Of course, it's easy to see why certain astrological signs, such as the Ram of Aries ♈, the Lion of Leo ♌, or the Archer of Sagittarius ♐, are *yang*. Aries ♈, the first sign of the Zodiac, is known for its pioneering ways. But why, you might wonder, is the Bull of Taurus ♉ not *yang*? Bull = masculine, right? Understanding how the attributes of each sign fit into *yin/yang* energy can deepen your understanding of *yin/yang* and how it can work for your health.

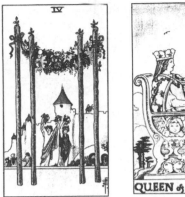
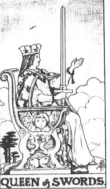

The 4 of Wands signals a yin approach of rest and recuperation, while the Queen of Swords signals action.

The Path of Yin

The nature of Taureans ♉ is that of dependability and sensuality. No one is more down to earth than a Taurus—or more immovable. Taurus is not the sign of direct action—in fact, the last thing a Bull likes is change. Taureans love the status quo more than anything else. And most of all, they seek harmony with all creatures on earth.

In the body, Taurus rules the neck and throat, which includes the thyroid and along with that the whole metabolic system. The energy of regulation, of keeping the body in balance, is *yin* energy.

Cancer ♋ is ruled by the Moon ☽. To understand how the Moon rules Cancer's *yin* polarity, remember from your third-grade science class that the Moon has no light source of its own; rather, it reflects light from the Sun ☉, and so it is with Cancer. Cancers reflect the moods and emotions of those around them. Crabs are all about feelings and nurturing. They are warm and sympathetic and highly sensitive. Body parts ruled by Cancer are the stomach and the breasts. Breasts are the ultimate in nurturing, the source of nourishment for tiny babies, the place to which we draw our loved ones when we hug them tight. The stomach is a receptive organ of the body—that which receives nourishment and sends it on to the rest of the body.

Virgo's ♍ image is the purest of *yin*—the Virgin. Virgo is about service, but just as much so, it is about wholeness. Virgos are intent on improving their health—and improving that of the world. Then, they will analyze it. They might not be the ones who start something—like an Aries ♈ or a Leo ♌—but they are definitely the ones who make sure it is done right. They might not be the first to create a vision, but they arc the first to see the sacred pattern in what is started. Virgos are introspective, and have a rich inner life. Sometimes, though, they may think too much.

So why isn't the Scorpion *yang?* It would seem like the sting of the Scorpion and the direct energy of *yang* go together. More than anything else, however, the sign of the Scorpion is about inner transformation—how the death of one life is the regeneration of the next. Scorpio ♏ is the night that becomes the day, the decaying leaves of late autumn that nourish the soil for the spring that lies ahead. Scorpio is the sign of rebirth—and most definitely *yin.* Note that Scorpio rules the genitals, the part of the body that is about regeneration of life. Scorpios have powerful imaginations and can have a rich dream life. They are tapped into their subconscious—the undercurrents of life. They speak fluently the language of nonverbal, nonmaterial world and can easily navigate the landscape of *yin.*

Capricorn ♑ is the *yin* of patience. A Capricorn, like no other sign, can bide her time, and she can be loyal to the end. A Capricorn is seeking security above all. Capricorn is *yin* because it rules the bones and teeth and all the connective tissue. This is the internal structure of the body, the alignment—more *yin.*

Like Scorpio, Pisces ♓ can dwell in the world of the imagination. They can be the last sign to have a grip on reality—a sheer escape. It is the sign of high intuition. A Pisces can be highly tuned to those around him. The symbol for Pisces is two crescent moons (very *yin*) linked together by a line—said to be the symbol for emotion and higher consciousness tied down to the material world.

The Path of Yang

Is there any doubt that the king of the jungle is a *yang* sign? Leos ♌ are dramatic, bold, exuberant. They are creative and strong—full of courage and long on pride. Leos are known for their willpower. When they want to make something happen, they can! Because this is a fixed sign, however, they can also get stuck in their habits. A lifetime of deeply ingrained health habits can be hard to turn around. Yet Leos can be the most intolerant of others who lack willpower. Leo the Lion is first and foremost about strength. The lion shows up in Tarot on the Strength card, too. When it comes to health, Leos promote strength; that's why this sign rules the back and the spine.

Gemini ♊ is a *yang* sign because it's a sign of motion. Geminis are known for their avid curiosity—yes, they'll be on the Internet, and they will be the ones asking the doctor all the questions, whether they are the patient or not. They are clever and adaptable—and not afraid to try something new.

Libra ♎ is one of the signs you might not immediately guess as *yang*. After all, Libra is about balance. Libra is the peacemaker. But Libra gets her *yang* from being the generator of a great deal of activity, much of it diplomacy. Libra is a thinker and is constantly in action. They are also very social creatures, the kind who are quick to form partnerships. Notice again, this is direct action, initiating and creating.

Sagittarians ♐ are energetic, daring, and adventurous. They are the first to sling the arrows of truth, and they can be very blunt and direct. They are the transformers—the ones who want to change the world with their truths.

The *yang* of Aquarius ♒ is that of the inventor. The drive toward invention is always stronger than something already known. Aquarians are idealistic and original. They are independent, and refuse to be categorized. An Aquarian is one of a kind, who sees the big picture and not the immediate scene. An Aquarian is always 10 years ahead and needs to remember to be in the present.

Here are the *yin* and *yang* of signs at a glance:

	Yin/Yang	Body Part	Yin/Yang Qualities
Aries ♈	*Yang*	Head, face, eyes, brain	Quick thinkers; quick to anger
Taurus ♉	*Yin*	Neck, throat	Inaction; slow metabolism
Gemini ♊	*Yang*	Hands, arms, shoulders, lungs	Curiosity; motion
Cancer ♋	*Yin*	Stomach, breasts	Feeling; nurturing
Leo ♌	*Yang*	Back, spine, heart	Strength; courage
Virgo ♍	*Yin*	Intestines, colon	Service; purity
Libra ♎	*Yang*	Kidneys, lower back, adrenal glands	Harmony; balance
Scorpio ♏	*Yin*	Genitals; urinary and reproductive system	Regeneration; the world of the subconscious
Sagittarius ♐	*Yang*	Liver, hips, thighs	Adventurer
Capricorn ♑	*Yin*	Bones, joints, knees	Patience
Aquarius ♒	*Yang*	Ankles, circulation	Inventor
Pisces ♓	*Yin*	Feet, immune system, hormonal system	High intuition

Astrology to Find Your Yin/Yang Balance

None of us is all *yin* or all *yang*. Your Sun ☉ sign is the beginning of identifying your personal *yin/yang* balance. To find your personal *yin/yang* balance, we use eight points in your astrological chart—your Sun ☉ sign; your Moon ☽ sign; your ascendant; and the planets Mercury ☿, Venus ♀, Mars ♂, Jupiter ♃, and Saturn ♄. Your three power point signs—Sun, Moon, and ascendant—will have more influence than the planets, but these others can help you fill in the whole *yin/yang* picture.

Knowing your personal *yin/yang* balance will give you clues to how you approach your health. If you are more predominantly *yang*, knowing that may help you understand you are the type of person who thrives once you are pointed on the path of direct action. And it will help you to know that you may resist during times when you must be receptive and let others guide you—to recognize when you need to be the receptor and when it's time for you to be pampered.

Let's take a look at the astrological birth chart of Deepak Chopra. What Chopra's chart reveals about *yin/yang* balance may give us clues as to why his life and work is to be a voice and vision bridging Eastern and Western medicine.

We have filled in this table to guide you in interpreting Chopra's *yin/yang* balance. As you can see, Chopra has five *yin* planets—many of them clustered in healing and transformative Scorpio ♏—and three *yang* planets. This indicates a subtle orientation to a *yin* approach to medicine, which may explain why after practicing conventional medicine for many years Chopra opened to seeking the balance in Eastern origins. His gentle yet powerful *yin* approach has transformed the way we think about the dynamic balance of mind, body, and spirit health.

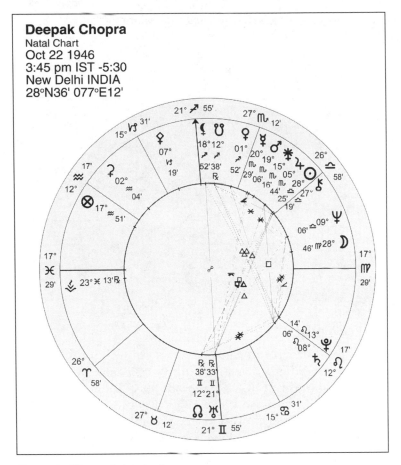

Deepak Chopra
Natal Chart
Oct 22 1946
3:45 pm IST -5:30
New Delhi INDIA
28°N36' 077°E12'

Deepak Chopra's birth chart.

Planet	Chopra's Astro Sign	Yin or Yang
Sun ☉	Libra ♎	*Yang*
Moon ☽	Virgo ♍	*Yin*
Mercury ☿	Scorpio ♏	*Yin*
Venus ♀	Sagittarius ♐	*Yang*
Mars ♂	Scorpio ♏	*Yin*
Jupiter ♃	Scorpio ♏	*Yin*
Saturn ♄	Leo ♌	*Yang*
Ascendant	Pisces ♓	*Yin*

Now, let's take a look at your *yin/yang* balance in your astrological birth chart.

Planet	Your Astro Sign	Yin or Yang
Sun ☉	_____	_____
Moon ☽	_____	_____
Mercury ☿	_____	_____
Venus ♀	_____	_____
Mars ♂	_____	_____
Jupiter ♃	_____	_____
Saturn ♄	_____	_____
Ascendant	_____	_____

Moon ☽ Time: Or When to Yin and When to Yang

Suppose your doctor just informed you that you will have to have a minor surgical procedure. When the surgery scheduler pronounces "8:30 A.M. Tuesday, the 26th," do you opt for a Tuesday morning, or do you push for a Monday so you can get it over with and get back to work by Thursday? Or do you say confidently, "Well, the Moon will be in Leo on Tuesday, and I need strength, so let's pick Tuesday."

Or maybe you are at peace with your upcoming surgery. It's the right thing to do, and you have a good doctor. So you may want to have your surgery during a *yin* time, submitting to an expert healer, the surgeon and her crew; then plan your recovery for a *yang* time, when you want to summon your energy to get recovery rolling.

The Moon ☽ goes through its cycle in 29½ days. Every 2½ days, it moves from one sign of the Zodiac to the next. Here's a quick look at how the Moon influences the energy of a day:

Moon In	Yin/Yang	Health Energy of the Day
Aries ♈	*Yang*	New beginnings; a time to push ahead
Taurus ♉	*Yin*	Steady course; getting bogged down
Gemini ♊	*Yang*	Time to talk; time to swing into motion

Moon In	Yin/Yang	Health Energy of the Day
Cancer ♋	Yin	Time for sympathy; moody; highly sensitive
Leo ♌	Yang	Courage; strength
Virgo ♍	Yin	Get organized; get critical; time to analyze; change your diet
Libra ♎	Yang	Equilibrium; fairness; time to see both sides of the question; but, indecisiveness
Scorpio ♏	Yin	Power; possessiveness; emotions run high; intensity runs your daily habits/exercise regimen
Sagittarius ♐	Yang	Restlessness; time for adventure; a time for truth, new discoveries; watch out for overindulgence
Capricorn ♑	Yin	Control; challenges; patience; businesslike, very serious in approach to health
Aquarius ♒	Yang	Invention; new ideas; independence; time to detach
Pisces ♓	Yin	Time to dream; time to intuit; time to imagine; escape

When the Moon ☽ is in Aries ♈, it's a good time to start a fitness plan or refine your nutritional plan, because Aries is about new beginnings. We definitely recommend avoiding scheduling a gut-wrenching session with your marriage therapist when the Moon is in Cancer ♋; that is, if you are a watery emotional type. Your feelings will just be too raw. However, if you are more left-brained and have trouble connecting with your feelings, the Moon in Cancer will help you. Know that when the Moon is in talkative Gemini ♊, it's the optimum time for analyzing your feelings. If you feel you are getting bogged down, that you aren't seeing any new, fresh ideas, check the Astrology reports—or the night sky. The Moon may be in Taurus ♉. Wait it out. Soon the Moon will be in Gemini, and you can swing into action then.

Yin and Yang Meet Tarot

So where does Tarot come into the picture with *yin/yang?* If you are already familiar with some of the archetypal figures and imagery in the

Tarot, you might be way ahead of us. The High Priestess of intuition is screaming "*yin,*" while the Emperor is definitely all "*yang.*" This exercise can help you bring the knowledge of *yin/yang* to your Tarot readings.

So let's get out the Tarot deck. We'll start with the Major Arcana. Lay out the 22 Major Arcana cards in order, starting with the Fool and ending with the World. One by one, look at each card. Does it feel *yin* or *yang* to you? Or does the card seem to tell the story of both *yin* and *yang*? Move *yin* cards to the left, *yang* cards to the right. If one seems like both, keep it in a center column.

Here's what happened when we did this exercise:

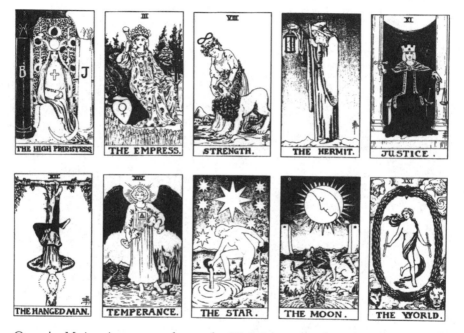

Our yin *Major Arcana cards are the High Priestess, the Empress, Strength, the Hermit, Justice, the Hanged Man, Temperance, the Star, the Moon, and the World.*

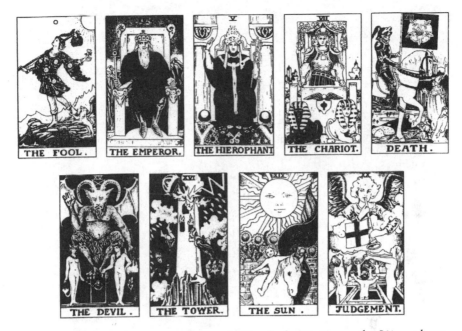

Our yang *Major Arcana cards are the Fool, the Emperor, the Hierophant, the Chariot, Death, the Devil, the Tower, the Sun, and Judgement.*

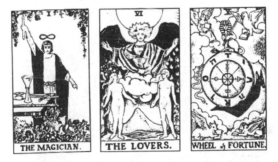

Our yin *and* yang *Major Arcana cards are the Magician, the Lovers, and the Wheel of Fortune.*

Remember, there are no right or wrong answers here. Your sort may be similar to ours, but then again it might not. The main aim of this exercise is to hone your intuition about *yin* and *yang* so you can learn to apply it yourself to your Tarot readings. It might be helpful to get out your Intuitive Arts notebook so you can make some notes about each card and its polarity.

As we went through the cards, we noted certain features—the main figure or figures on the card, its imagery, colors, and symbols, landscapes, and heavenly bodies. Start with the first card in your *yin* column. What about it made you decide it represented *yin* energies?

We picked the High Priestess. Here are some of our notes:

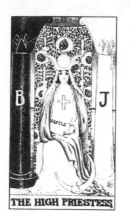

High Priestess = *yin*

intuitive

receptive

pomegranates (myth of Persephone; image of fecundity)

unseen

mystery

hidden truths

crescent moon

beneath the surface

insight

inner listening

For *yang*, one of our picks was the Chariot. Here are some of our notes:

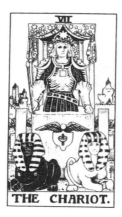

The Chariot = *yang*

success

conquest

will

authority

fortitude

triumph

perseverance

inner strength

Note that we picked some cards as the embodiment of both energies. The Magician, for instance, is pointing one hand to heaven (*yang*), the other to earth (*yin*). He also has symbols from all four Minor Arcana suits set out before him on the table where he is about to do his work. This suggests well-roundedness. A figure 8 floats over his head like a halo. This is the symbol of a continuum, two halves of a whole. The Magician represents the ability to turn our ideas (the unborn of *yin*) to something tangible (*yang*).

The Lovers card also represents dualities. The imagery is of a woman and a man coming together. But notice that behind her is the Tree of Knowledge (cognitive knowing, or *yang* knowing), while behind him are the 12 signs of the Zodiac (intuitive knowing, or *yin* knowing). He represents conscious mind and reason (*yang*), while she represents the subconscious and emotion (*yin*).

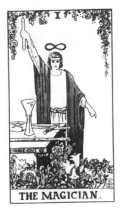

The Magician = *yin/yang*

Yin

pointing to earth

receptive

fullness, open vessel, figure 8, symbol of continuum

flowers

cup (emotion)

white lilies (purity)

Yang

pointing to heaven

unleashing power

creativity

all the tools of his trade are before him; he is about to take direct action

red roses (passion)

Time to Yin, Time to Yang

While the Major Arcana are Tarot's destiny cards—who am I, and who I am meant to be—the Minor Arcana are the day-to-day cards. They are often called the free-will cards, because they are about the ability to choose. When these cards show up, they are about the choices you have made or will make.

Each suit of the Minor Arcana symbolizes an area of life and carries a *yin/yang* energy:

Tarot Suit	Keyword	Yin/Yang Energy
Wands	Enterprise	*Yang*
Cups	Emotion	*Yin*
Swords	Action	*Yang*
Pentacles	Resources	*Yin*

Wands. Wands represent ambition and the ability to grow and develop. Think of a magic wand: The realm of Wands is the realm of creation and ideas. They are about manifesting dreams into material life.

Cups. Cups represent how we perceive our emotions. Think of the cup of communion: This is the place for the heart, for finding your feelings and being aware of others' feelings. The Cups are associated with water, a symbol of the unconscious mind and intuition. The Cups are the vessel for all of our emotional connections.

Swords. Swords are not only about doing battle, though they can be symbolic of strife or aggression. Mainly, Swords are about action and mental ability, about how we think, how we use logic and reasoning.

Pentacles. Pentacles represent the currency of life, the flow of how we do business. They are the cards of the material world, of money, possessions, and earthly things—the resources we use to manifest our desires. They often show up when you have a question about security.

Use Tarot to Find Your Yin/Yang Balance

A Seven-Card Tarot Spread can help you pinpoint your *yin/yang* equation. As you shuffle, you may want to meditate on a broad question such as, *"What is the picture of my health?"* to gain insight into which areas may be out of *yin/yang* balance. Or you may have a specific illness, and the question may be, *"How do I equip myself to overcome this condition?"* or *"How am I naturally equipped to restore my health?"* But no matter how you focus it, the central question of this spread is, *"Who am I?"* from a *yin/yang* place of balance.

We chose a Seven-Card Spread for this big-picture question because this spread is effective for times when you need more than a "yes" or "no" answer, when you need deep knowing and divine wisdom. In this spread, the first two cards represent the past. The next three cards represent the present, and the last two cards represent the future.

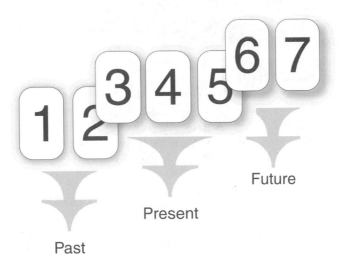

Future

Present

Past

The Seven-Card Spread. The first two cards represent the past, the next three cards represent the present, and the last two cards represent the future.

Diane's question for Arlene: "What is the focus of my health now?"

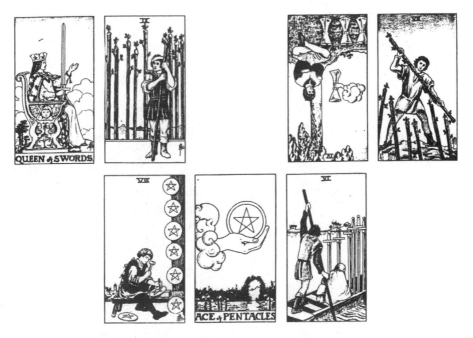

Arlene's reading for Diane.

The Past: Queen of Swords, 9 of Wands. These indicate Diane has been very aware of health issues before they got out of hand. Both cards indicate a well-prepared person and both are *yang,* indicating Diane is proactive about her health.

The Present: 8 of Pentacles, Ace of Pentacles, 6 of Swords. Diane is working toward maintaining good health, possibly by working out and boning up on health issues. A new beginning in her health regimen is revitalizing her energy. The 6 of Swords shows Diane's ability to traverse the rocky waters of health, or possibly a depression she has experienced and released. Way to go!

The Future: 4 of Cups R, 7 of Wands. These cards signal the return of hope and happiness to Diane's health. The 4 of Cups reversed says a lot about emotionally "getting into it," accepting that she needs to keep the discipline of a routine. The last card suggests that at times, Diane will feel intimidated by the task of keeping up with her exercise routine. But Diane will maintain a good balance between rest and action. As she learns more about her health, she will be able to face what might threaten her health and not be so afraid of it. After this reading, Diane seemed empowered to participate in seeking knowledge and maintaining discipline about her health.

A Science of Opposites: Yin/Yang and Ayurveda

Ayurveda is a Sanskrit word, deriving from two roots: *ayur* means life; *veda* means knowledge. So ayurveda is the knowledge of life. Ayurveda believes that every human being is created from pure cosmic consciousness from two energies. *Purusha* is pure consciousness, unexpressed and unknowable, the latent force of nature or choiceless passive awareness. *Prakriti* is manifestation, creation, the principle of desire. *Prakriti* is choiceful active consciousness. Like *yin/yang,* ayurveda is about healthful balance of polarities.

Ayurvedic practitioners work with a system broken down into 10 pairs of opposites. These pairs are used in identifying tendencies and imbalances in diet, skin tone, emotional constitution, and activity. In the next chapter, we take a peek at how ayurveda applies these principles of opposites to diet.

Heavy	Light
Sharp	Dull, slow
Hot	Cold
Oily	Dry

Dense/solid	Liquid
Rough	Smooth
Hard	Soft
Gross	Subtle
Mobile	Static
Sticky	Clear

Ayurvedic medicine treats the patient (*rogi*) and the disease (*roga*). One does not exist without the other. It's another *yin/yang* relationship: In every patient who has a disease, there is a human being; in every disease, there is also health. In conventional Western medicine, patients in a hospital are often referred to by disease or condition: "The acute appendicitis in Room 314." The team of doctors and nurses focus on the disease. But ayurveda sees that aspects of health exist alongside the disease in any patient, and it uses that reservoir of health in restoring balance and eliminating the disease.

Know Thyself, Heal Thyself

As we wrote this chapter, we learned more about ourselves, too. Perhaps you are a workaholic Virgo ♍, and reading through this chapter made you think about ways to not work so hard; or maybe you're a Capricorn ♑, and you realized you need to take better care of your bones and teeth. In seeking insight through Astrology, Tarot, and Psychic Intuition, we often receive information that resonates with the deep knowing we already possess inside us. You know your body, your mind, and your spirit more than anyone else. Are you the ocean or the beach? The cloud or the rain? The night or the day? Are you the High Priestess or the Chariot's driver? Are you the Aquarian Water-Bearer or Taurus's Bull? Is it time to ascend or descend, to wait and receive or start and swing into motion, to expand your life and create something new or contract, pull in, and reflect? Take a moment to make a few notes here or in your Intuitive Arts notebook.

_____

_____

_____

_____

Knowing your *yin/yang* balance is the beginning of healthy mind, body, and spirit synergy. It is the beginning of creating harmony. You will learn to tap into your natural ways of healing. And you will learn to accept that disharmony is part of the process. The power of the body, mind, and spirit to heal itself is amazing. Trust in its potential and move toward your centering balance.

chapter 3

Health Is Elemental

Fire and rain
Power points: The Elements and Astrology
Inspiration rising
Tarot and the Elements
The Chinese Elements
Celebrating your Elemental strengths
Knowing your Elemental weaknesses
Ayurveda and the Elements

The four Elements—Fire, Earth, Air, and Water—are the essence of health and vitality. By combining Astrology's power points, Tarot, and Psychic Intuition, you can identify your Elemental Health Signature, which is as unique as the whorls on your fingertips that define your fingerprints. Each of the Tarot's Major Arcana cards, and each of its four Minor Arcana suits, connects with an Element, so we'll let the imagery of the Tarot guide us in connecting the Elements to the Elemental chemistry that is uniquely you. We show you how the Elements can put you in touch with how much you already know intuitively about your health now. Knowing how the Elements influence your health can be the key to developing the good habits and stress-relieving techniques that can free you from chronic problems— or head off problems that, if left unattended, may come up later in life. By identifying your Elemental Health Signature, you can learn to maintain the optimal balance of body, mind, and spirit.

Fire and Rain

Walk into a hospital lobby, and you'll likely see a directory guiding you to various specialists for different parts of the body: gastronomical, vascular, neurological, obstetrics. Just as there are ear, nose, and throat doctors; heart doctors; and baby-delivering doctors, the Elements represent specialties and identify vital energy forces of the body, mind, and spirit. Let's get to know the Elements and how they work in balance for optimal health.

All of the Elements are connected to astrological signs. Let's take a look:

Fire	Earth	Air	Water
Aries ♈	Taurus ♉	Gemini ♊	Cancer ♋
Leo ♌	Virgo ♍	Libra ♎	Scorpio ♏
Sagittarius ♐	Capricorn ♑	Aquarius ♒	Pisces ♓

An Unforgettable Fire

Fire represents the life force of the body. It relates to blood, which brings nutrients to all cells in the body. Fire is our passion for life, our drive and energy and power. Fire is the spirit that infuses our flesh, the light within our hearts, the spark in our eyes. Fire can also be heat, as in the metabolic process of burning calories. Does this mean Fire signs—Aries ♈, Leo ♌, and Sagittarius ♐—have a higher metabolism and therefore have no problem working off calories? ("Yes!" we can hear all of you Fire signs saying.) Unfortunately, this is not true for Carolyn, an Archer, but she is definitely passionate about all things in life, with a constant thirst for new knowledge and new experiences and enough energy to keep up with her 3-year-old boy/girl twins—and that definitely burns calories.

The Rare Earth

Earth is about being grounded. It is the essential underlying structure of the body. Earth is the matrix, or the skeleton. So while Fire is the blood, Earth is the bones. Earth holds it all together. Earth is also about DNA, the basic building blocks of the body. Earth sign people—Taurus ♉, Virgo ♍, and Capricorn ♑—are very sensual, very tactile, because they are always more aware of where their feet are planted. They may love to walk barefoot on the beach, feeling the sand between their toes, or turn a spade in the rich, dark soil of a vegetable garden. If you have a strong Earth presence in your Elemental Health Signature (read on to find out!), you will be more aware of your fingers tapping the keyboard as you sit at the computer, because you constantly want to be connected with the physical world. This natural body awareness gives you a built-in advantage: Earth Element people tend to take good care of their health. But you also might have a lower tolerance for pain.

Good Vibrations

Air, of course, is about breath. The Air Element relates to your lungs and your voice box. When your Air Element is optimum, it's about resonance—the rich vibration of sound health. Air feeds your cells with oxygen, but it also feeds your mental power. How do your thoughts affect your body? Are you a power thinker? What beliefs influence how you experience pain or how you heal? Can you easily transcend pain? You may have a strong Air Element influence in your Elemental Health Signature. Air is definitely something you want to cultivate on the day you're having dental surgery. If you have a strong Air influence, you may excel in personal expression. For instance, Arlene has two Air signs in her astrological power points (more about those coming up) and she thrives on music, art, or anything that requires a creative vision. Thinking, envisioning, and analyzing are all important to the Air signs—Gemini ♊, Libra ♎, and Aquarius ♒.

Like a River Flows

Water is the flow of the body, but also of the heart. It represents our feelings toward ourselves and others. Water signs—Cancer ♋, Scorpio ♏, and Pisces ♓—and those with dominant Water presence in their Elemental Health Signatures are more expressive of their emotions and are susceptible to being swept up in the emotion of the moment. Yes, they always cry at weddings. Water is necessary as the transport of nutrients to healthy cells and is essential for promoting harmony between all organs and systems of the body. Water, too, is needed to flush out wastes. If you have ever had a massage, you may have been advised to drink plenty of water after everything got loosened up. Your massage therapist may be like Carolyn's, who provides a bottle of spring water with each massage. Sometimes Carolyn hears from her massage therapist that the muscles in her neck and shoulders are "crunchy"—too much Fire trapped in there. That is where the heat and soreness come from; the waste has gotten trapped in muscle tissue and needs to be flushed out. Water also relates to the hormonal system. So don't say you're hormonal—just say, "My Water Element is strong today," as you sob into a tissue.

Drawing upon what we learned about *yin* and *yang* in Chapter 2, we can understand also that each Element has balancing qualities. Each Element flows into another: Water absorbs into Earth, descending, becoming material. Fire ascends, condensing Water into Air.

So that's a taste of how the Elements embody us. Here's a chart with Elemental keywords that you can refer to as we go along.

Fire	Earth	Air	Water
Life force	Structure of the body	Breath	Flow of the body
Blood	Bone	Voice	Emotions
Passion	Groundedness	Mental power	Hormones
Power	Touch	Thoughts	Harmony
Drive, ambition	Sensual	Beliefs	Replenishment of cells
Enthusiasm	DNA	Mind over matter	Sensitivity
Strength	Fertility	Lightness of being	Pregnancy
Metabolic process	Abundance	Vision	Nurturing, empathy

Power Points of Your Elemental Health Signature

Carolyn's three-year-old son likes to play that he is "throwing fire" at the monsters, the sharp-tooth dinosaurs, or whatever threat is at hand. This is a metaphor for his body's defenses. And yes, he's a Leo ♌—a Fire sign—so that explains his weapon of choice.

How can you know what defenses your body naturally has to remove disease and pain and restore health? Whether you are looking to rebalance a tendency toward depression, manage chronic pain, or just steel yourself through a rocky life transition, the Elements can help center and rejuvenate your body, mind, and spirit. Let's look at Astrology's Elemental power points, the core of your Elemental Health Signature.

Use the three power points of your astrological birth chart—your Sun ☉ sign, your Moon ☽ sign, and your ascendant, or rising sign.

Power Point	Energics	Action
Sun ☉	Self, essence, life spirit, creativity, willpower	Explores
Moon ☽	Emotions, instincts, unconscious, past memories	Senses
Ascendant	Outward appearance, public persona, body	Displays

Knowing your personal astrological power points is a must to identify the strengths and weaknesses of your whole self—your integrated body, mind, and spirit. Once you know your power point strengths and their vulnerable flip sides, you can cultivate the habits that keep you at optimum health and use potential weaknesses as a barometer to know when you are asking too much of your body. To identify your Astrological Elemental power points, find the Sun ☉, Moon ☽, and ascendant in your birth chart and note each planet's sign placement in your chart, as well as that sign's Element.

	Arlene	Carolyn	You
Sun ☉ sign	Aquarius ♒/Air	Sagittarius ♐/Fire	_____
Moon ☽ sign	Gemini ♊/Air	Aquarius ♒/Air	_____
Ascendant	Pisces ♓/Water	Virgo ♍/Earth	_____

Arlene is an Aquarius Sun ♒ ☉, Gemini Moon ♊ ☽, and Pisces ♓ rising. That gives Arlene two Air Elements and one Water Element as her astrological power points. Arlene has always had trouble defending her body against airborne attackers—pollen, dust, cat dander, you name it. Her respiratory system—sinuses, ears, throat—have always been sensitive. With the Water Element, Pisces ♓, Arlene has experienced problems with hormones, her immune system, and the water level in her body at different times in her life. She doesn't really like to drink a lot of water, and did she suffer until she got it that she needed to do that! Her lymph nodes and other immune system indicators got blocked and—boom!—upper respiratory infection.

To see more about how this works, let's look at the birth chart for Oprah Winfrey, who has inspired many with her commitment to healthy body, mind, and spirit.

Power Point	Astro Sign	Element
Sun ☉	Aquarius ♒	Air
Moon ☽	Sagittarius ♐	Fire
Ascendant	Virgo ♍	Earth

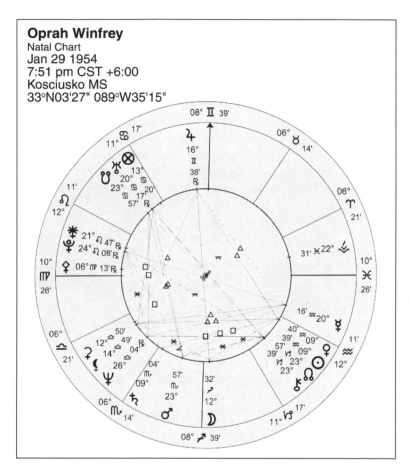

Oprah Winfrey's birth chart.

Oprah is well-balanced, with three of the Elements in her power points. This isn't that surprising, as she's dedicated her life and her spirit to balance. As someone who has dealt with weight, body image, and emotional issues, Oprah offers herself as a strong voice to temper the barrage of negative cultural messages we receive about our bodies. In the pages of her magazine, *O, The Oprah Magazine* (August 2002), she invited readers to celebrate their bodies—even the flaws—by writing a love letter to their most despised or neglected body part. That same issue featured portraits of women celebrating their favorite body part—a sleek muscular back, shapely calves, a round derriere. All of these women are beautiful, but not in the typical fashion model way—more like the women in your own circle of friends.

With her Sun ☉ in Aquarius ♒ and her Moon ☽ in Sagittarius ♐, Oprah is an enthusiastic humanitarian. Add Virgo ♍ rising and you see Oprah has a strong tendency toward self-improvement and refinement. Rising Virgins are working on developing a deeper understanding of their contribution to contemporary culture. Once they understand their own sacred work—as Oprah has—they can co-create with the spiritual patterns of the universe. This may explain why Oprah has really hit her stride at midlife.

Tarot and the Elements: In the Cards

Now that you know your astrological power points, let's add Tarot to complete your Elemental Health Signature. Each Major Arcana card is associated with an astrological sign(s) and, so, with its Element. Using the following table, identify a Major Arcana card(s) that corresponds with the astrological sign and Element of your power points. Meditate upon the imagery and significance of the card to deepen your understanding and complete your Elemental Health Signature.

For Oprah, we've chosen the Star for her Aquarius Sun ♒ ☉, the Chariot for her Sagittarius Moon ♐ ☽, and the High Priestess for her Virgo ♍ ascendant. We especially like the High Priestess as she brings the fourth Element, Water, as well as Earth, to complete Oprah's Elemental power.

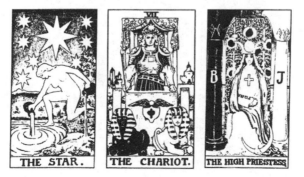

Oprah's astrological Elemental power points expressed through Tarot's Major Arcana reveal her Elemental Health Signature.

Tarot Card	Astrological Sign(s)	Element	Significance
The Fool	Aries ♈	Fire	Initiation, adventure, but also a tendency to leap without looking
Magician	Aries ♈	Fire	Creating magic, passion
High Priestess	Pisces ♓, Virgo ♍	Water and Earth	Senses heightened to a higher level of psychic awareness
Empress	Taurus ♉, Libra ♎	Earth and Air	Earth mother; creating abundance, beauty, comfort, nourishment, security
Emperor	Aries ♈, Scorpio ♏	Fire and Water	Leadership, power, mastery
Hierophant	Taurus ♉	Earth	Constancy, conformity; educator; consensus-builder
The Lovers	Gemini ♊	Air	Partnership; dualities; making choices, seeking balance
Chariot	Sagittarius ♐	Fire	The health card; victory over health problems; stamina; personal power
Strength	Leo ♌	Fire	Creating courage, inner/physical strength
Hermit	Virgo ♍	Earth	Seeking inner truth; sharing sacred wisdom
Wheel of Fortune	Aquarius ♒, Taurus ♉, Leo ♌, Scorpio ♏	Air, Earth, Fire, and Water	Attuning yourself to the natural ebb and flow of life; finding constancy within the mystery of life
Justice	Libra ♎	Air	Seeing life from both sides; achieving balance; seeking what is fair and honorable

Tarot Card	Astrological Sign(s)	Element	Significance
Hanged Man	Pisces ♓	Water	Sacrifice and release; the art of letting go; relinquishing the material for the spiritual
Death	Scorpio ♏	Water	Old things become new again; regeneration; rejuvenation; the phoenix rising from the ashes
Temperance	Cancer ♋	Water	Tempering the changeability of life with patience, adaptability; balancing emotions (water) and logic (earth)
The Devil	Capricorn ♑	Earth	Surmounting the temptations of the material world; releasing your darkest fears
The Tower	Aquarius ♒	Air	Innovative change; bold awakening
The Star	Aquarius ♒	Air	Hope for a better tomorrow; courage; inspiration
The Moon	Cancer ♋	Water	Psychic attunement to feelings in the world at large; the ability to "see" and "feel" conditions occurring that can manifest the emotional nature
The Sun	Leo ♌	Fire	Inner peace; contentment about life; drive; optimism
Judgement	Scorpio ♏	Water	Awakening emotions to the third eye; the ability to connect feelings to a higher level; the ability to attain epiphany; revealing of the mysteries of life; to know, to integrate, to accept change
The World	Capricorn ♑	Earth	Triumph, attainment, fulfillment

Your Everyday Elemental Health Tarot Spread

Each suit of Tarot's Minor Arcana matches up with an Element.

Fire	Earth	Air	Water
Wands	Pentacles	Swords	Cups

With the Minor Arcana cards, every day carries an Elemental Health Signature. Find out your daily Elemental Health Signature with a simple Four-Card Tarot Spread. For this exercise, you use the Minor Arcana cards only, so go through your Tarot deck now and set aside the 22 Major Arcana cards. As you shuffle the remaining 56 cards, meditate on finding out the day's Elemental Health Signature. It is helpful to articulate it as a thought, or even say it out loud: "Show me my health/ energy level today." When you feel ready, cut the deck into four separate decks. They don't have to be even. Then turn each of the stacks over. The cards on the bottom of each stack represent the day's Elemental Health Signature.

All kinds of combinations are possible. You may get four different Elements or two of the same with two different ones. If you get two or three of the same, that Element will dominate the day, while the other two will keep you balanced. A day with four different Elements will be very balanced. A day with all four Elements in one suit is definitely one you should prepare for—that Elemental influence will be *strong!*

Out in the Elements: Your Connection to the Natural World

Ancient Chinese medicine has always recognized our connection with the Elements and the natural world. In traditional Chinese medicine, there are five Elements—Fire, Wood, Metal, Earth, and Water—that represent agents of change and reaction in the body. Each of these connects with Astrology, Tarot, and the seasons.

As the seasons correspond to the Elements, they correspond to the essential movements of life. The more in tune you are with the natural movement of life, the more in harmony your body, mind, and spirit will be with all of the forces of life on our planet. The Elements in Chinese medicine also are part of a *Shen*, or nourishing cycle, in which each Element has a Mother-Son relationship: Water nourishes Wood; Wood fuels Fire; Fire makes Earth (ashes); Earth yields Metal; and Metal produces Water (condensation). Each Element has a tempering effect on another, and this is called the *Ko* cycle, said to be a Grandmother-Son relationship: Water extinguishes Fire; Fire melts Metal; Metal cuts Wood; Wood can contain Earth; and Earth absorbs Water.

Chinese Element	Wood	Fire	Earth	Metal	Water
Season	Beginning of **spring**—rising creativity	Early **summer**—joy, laughter, partnership	Late **summer**—bittersweet, a time of relinquishing expectations, becoming more grounded	**Fall**—letting go, a time of awe and respect	**Winter**—quiet, going within, cultivating a deeper wisdom
Tarot	Wands	Wands	Pentacles	Swords	Cups
Element	Fire	Fire	Earth	Air	Water
Organ of Influence	Gall-bladder	Tongue, intestines	Spleen, pancreas, mouth	Lungs, respiratory system	Kidney, urinary tract, inner-ear balance

Let's go deeper and see how the cycles of life can work for you. For instance, Water is winter. Winter is a time of gestation, of waiting and not yet seeing the new life that will emerge in spring. So it is a time of unknowing, of quiet, of going within. In winter, we store up our energy to await a time of new growth. This can mean a storing up of wisdom. With the quiet of a new-fallen snow—a quiet that can surpass any quiet you have ever known—it is also a time of deep listening—to our inner voice, to the pulse of the natural world.

Now, Carolyn was born on the winter solstice, so the time of winter is very comforting for her. As a writer, it is easy for her to slip into her contemplative side. On the day she wrote this, the Sandia Mountains in Albuquerque were behind a massive white curtain of snow, as the days on the calendar marched toward winter solstice. With 300-plus days of sunshine each year in Albuquerque, these days are rare, even in winter. So Carolyn found the Elements around her very invigorating. But for most of us, in our busy-busy-busy, information-overload, touch-tone express, automatic overdrive lives, this time of winter—of slowing down, listening deeply, and going within—is one we often resist. Maybe that's why our culture insists on such a swirl of activity around the holidays. And maybe that's why flu season follows right after the tinsel is packed away, the tree is recycled, and the sweaters that didn't fit are exchanged. Your body, mind, and spirit demand that you slow down.

Once you know your Elemental Health Signature and learn more about how to use Astrology and the Tarot to guide you through changes, you will no longer resist but instead know that you can embrace these movements of the seasons and the Elements in your life. A daily Elemental Tarot reading can signal you to these movements of the natural world around you. It can signal you to cultivate the time of laughter—early summer—in your life. It can also point you to when it's time to start letting go of people, places, or practices that are no longer working for your optimal health and benefit.

The Wheel of Fortune card in the Tarot illustrates this quite well because it has four signs: Aquarius ≈, Taurus ♉, Leo ♌, and Scorpio ♏. Each of these signs represents a season: Aquarius is winter, Taurus is spring, Leo is summer, and Scorpio is autumn. When the Wheel of Fortune comes up, you receive a strong message to embrace the natural cycle of life. Notice also that each sign represents a different Element: Aquarius is Air, Taurus is Earth, Leo is Fire, and Scorpio is Water. So this card can indicate a harmony between the Elements.

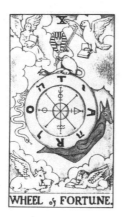

Tarot's Wheel of Fortune embraces the Elements and their seasons.

We're Wired: Our Connection to Ourselves

Traditional Chinese medicine relates the systems of the body to meridians, or a series of energy pathways through the body. Think of a meridian as a fiber-optic cable running through your body transmitting vital energy from one area to another. Acupuncture points are distributed along these meridians. There are more than 400 acupoints. Oriental medicine practitioners believe by getting the proper amount of energy to the proper place in the body, the body's natural healing process is stimulated. Did you know the body produces natural painkillers, anti-inflammatory agents, and disease-fighting elements? Acupuncture activates those by getting vital energy forces back in balance.

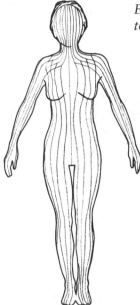

Energy pathways connect to the Elements.

The Elements come into play in how acupuncture works with the meridians. For instance, in the *yin* meridians, the *Ying* (spring) point belongs to the Fire Element, which means it releases heat from its related meridian or organ system.

For many years, Carolyn has gone to a massage therapist who uses Psychic Intuition. The massage therapist emphasizes breath awareness in her practice and activates her knowledge of the meridians and reflexology to point Carolyn's attention toward whatever is out of balance. The therapist often concentrates a lot of time at the beginning of the session on foot massage, because our feet have many meridian points. Starting on these meridians releases a lot of the blocked energy. If you practice yoga, you probably also know about the role of flexion—flexing your feet—as you breathe through a pose, pushing energy out through your heel. Sure enough, at the end of a session, the massage therapist sends

Carolyn out the door with instructions such as: "Drink raspberry-leaf tea for one week," or "Try this Bach's flower essence." With just a little knowledge of the meridians and a lot of listening to your body, you can employ these methods, too. If you have had a massage, you probably already know which parts of your body really need attention and which parts "react" and are activated by the stimulus of massage.

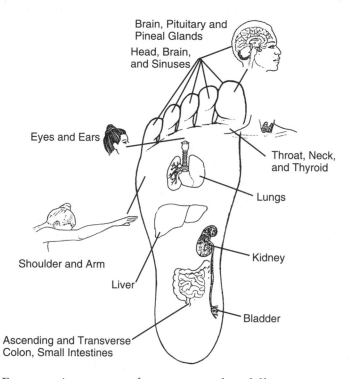

Energy points on your feet correspond to different areas of the body.

When Carolyn was pregnant with the twins, her therapist avoided massaging the area on her inside heel. Why? Because the energy meridian there is connected with the uterus, and massaging there could have activated premature labor contractions. Now, knowing that piece about massaging your inside heel can come in handy if you are: (1) having terrible premenstrual syndrome or are (2) 10 days past full gestation, big as a house, and thinking 24 hours or so of screaming pain would be better than being pregnant another minute. The remedy might be as simple as massaging your inside heel.

Tarot, too, can point you to blocked energy centers when a card is reversed. But the following exercise is more fun, and we definitely recommend you try it. It requires making a date for a foot massage with someone who loves you well. First, you need almond oil and a reflexology diagram. (Detailed diagrams are available for less than $5 on the Internet. Try www.aboutreflexology.com.) Then add some candles and a little soft music, a fire in the fireplace. You set the scene. Remember, this is a fact-finding mission. Ask your massage partner to work his or her way around the bottom of your foot with two thumbs circulating in clockwise and counterclockwise motion. Your part is to close your eyes and empty your mind. Breathe in through your nose and out through your mouth. Notice as he or she works across your feet which points resist the pressure. Notice if you experience pain or activate energy in other parts of your body as well. Did you get a twinge of pain in your shoulder, a stab of pain in your knee? Does your stomach gurgle? Your pinkie finger twitch? Notice, too, the points that welcome the pressure.

Balancing the Elements: Celebrating Your Strengths

As you begin to work with *yin/yang* as you learned in Chapter 2 and your essential Elements as you're learning here, you develop a sense of your body, mind, and spirit strengths and weaknesses. Celebrate your strengths and cultivate the habits that will make these resources you can rely on. Know that probably you have gravitated already to certain foods, types of exercise, and soul-enriching practices that boost your health. A friend of Carolyn's who has a background in holistic health once told her that her affinity for dry red wine and strong coffee came naturally—a Fire sign's way of shoring up the body's natural cancer-fighting abilities. Carolyn's 3-year-old daughter with astrological Elemental power points of Fire-Earth-Water *loves* capers and pickles. She can down a third of a jar of capers in one sitting. (We can only imagine what she will crave when she's in *her* last month of pregnancy!) Carolyn believes her daughter's affinity for that taste is something that she seeks intuitively to thrive, though it is not a taste Carolyn enjoys!

Once you have identified your Elemental Health Signature, you can begin to celebrate your strengths. Is there something that really just does it for you? Is there something you have always relied on to elevate your energy or lift your spirits? You have probably intuitively gravitated toward that food or that exercise. Take the time to celebrate the way your body takes care of you. After a good workout at the health club, the instructor often will say to give your body a hug of appreciation for trying so hard. Develop some affirmations that you can practice every day. A good resource for those is the Institute for Transformation, www.transformation.org, which can send you an e-mail affirmation every day. The power of hearing it in your own voice is immense. Try saying this one aloud.

I am a confident, radiant, successful person. I can afford to be very generous with my energy.

Or use the Tarot to guide you. If the Strength card comes up, and you have shown courage lately in facing surgery or illness or stress, then heed that, and affirm your strength.

I am filled with courage to face any seeming obstacles that come my way. I know that my Higher Being is greater than any problem, and we will triumph.

Start a book of affirmations or a special section for them in your Intuitive Arts notebook. At the beginning, write your natural power points, listing your body's natural strengths. These two steps are the beginning of embracing your body with lifelong affection and respect. Arlene and Carolyn had fun making up their list of natural power points—and we learned something, too! We have left some space for you to fill in yours.

	Arlene	Carolyn	You
Natural power foods	Chicken	Yogurt smoothies	_____
	Natural yogurt	Water, lots of water	_____
	Orange juice	Vine-ripened tomatoes	_____
	Pineapple	Leafy greens	_____
	Cranberries	Red bell peppers	_____
	Salmon	Berries	_____
	Coffee	Lemongrass glass noodles	_____
	Almonds	Salmon	_____
	Apricots	Cilantro	_____
	Basil	Basil	_____
	Tomatoes	Arugula	_____

	Arlene	Carolyn	You
	Garlic	Strong coffee	_____
	Corn on the cob	Anything with caramel	_____
	Lemongrass soup	Chocolate	_____
	Rice	Curry	_____
Natural power exercises	Hot tub/sauna	Studio cycling/ outdoor cycling	_____
	Gardening		_____
	Beach hiking	Hiking in the woods	_____
	Modern dance;	Walking by the river	_____
	water aerobics	Nia (dance/movement to world beat music)	_____
Natural soul-soothers	Walking miles	My children	_____
	Friends	Yoga	_____
	Hot bath/sauna	Travel	_____
	Driving	Writing/journaling	_____
	Massage	Prayer	_____
	Gatherings	Music	_____
	Barbecues	Mountains	_____
	Photography	Bubble baths	_____
	Cats	Fire in the fireplace	_____
	Fragrant herbs	Hot stone massage	_____
	Intuitive Arts	Candles	_____

Got Fire? Got Water? Shoring Up Your Weak Points

Now, remember the massage therapist who practices Psychic Intuition? It often came up when Carolyn went to her that Carolyn has too much Air and Fire—a lot of intellectual power but not enough grounding. That means spending more time gardening, turning the earth, or going for long walks or walking around barefoot on the brick floor. Because Carolyn has a Fire Sun ☉ sign, it often came up that her diet is too acidic and she needs to balance it with alkaline foods. Sure enough, Carolyn—who loves tomatoes, orange juice, and coffee—wouldn't know an alkaline food if it dropped out of the sky and knocked her on the head. The massage therapist advised her to go out and buy some umeboshi paste—a paste of pickled plums often used in Asian cooking. Did we say pickled? Well, needless to say, Carolyn didn't like the taste. It sat in her refrigerator for a year until she moved to a new house. But the massage therapist meant well. Sometimes we find it easier than other times to play against our natural tendencies to shore up our weaknesses.

One way to tune in to what's out of balance in your body, mind, and spirit is to look more deeply at the four cards of your daily Elemental Health Tarot Spread, posing the question, *"Show me my energy level and vitality today. Show me what's out of balance."* Often, you will find you have too much of one Element, not enough of another. When that is revealed to you, let it inform your decision to restore the body's natural balance. Too much Air, not enough Water can be too much thinking, a separation of the head from the heart. The extreme of that can be depression, as can the combination of too much Earth, not enough Fire. Too much Earth in the day's energy can make a person slow and methodical. Moreover, if you have a too-strong Earth Element in your astrological power points, you may either be obsessed with health and body image, or you may care less. Arlene says she rarely sees the in-between. It's always to the max with a too-much Earth person. To temper too much Fire in the day, seek more Earth or Water. Ground yourself by touching earth, working in the garden, or petting your animals. Or go for a swim. To temper too much Water, seek Earth practices to ground yourself or Air to lift yourself out of emotions that are overwhelming you. Remember, as you are seeking out that balance, that Water and Earth are the cooling elements; Fire and Air are the warming elements.

Ayurveda and the Elements

Ayurveda separates food guidelines into three groups that match three of the elements—Air, Water, and Fire. There are three main types—Vata (Air), Pitta (Fire), and Kapha (Water)—and four combination types. An ayurvedic diet enhances the natural tendencies of each type and restores imbalances. The thinking behind ayurvedic diet is that there is no one-prescription-fits-all diet; rather, it individualizes foods to optimize nutrition based on your constitution and any imbalances that may exist.

To find out more about your type, there are many ayurvedic books that instruct in self-identification, or you may visit an ayurvedic practitioner. You may, however, immediately recognize yourself in one of these types. Knowing your ayurvedic type can help you understand your body's basic structure and function, as well as any disposition to certain types of diseases.

We adapt this breakdown from *The New Whole Foods Encyclopedia* (Penguin/Arkana, 1999) with a little help from Michael Dick, ayurvedic consultant at The Ayurvedic Institute in Albuquerque. As you read down through the three types, remember *yin/yang's* pairs of opposites from Chapter 2. For example, Pitta types tend to be oily, hot, and light, so they need a diet that is cool, slightly dry, and somewhat heavy.

Vata: Air

A Vata, or Air type, may be someone who is quick moving, fleet of foot, active, and energetic. A Vata may think more creatively and intuitively. The weaknesses of a Vata type are all degenerative. Weak circulation may mean cold hands. Too much energy and strong intellect can go hand and hand with worry, fear, and anxiety. Vata people flourish with a warming, grounding diet emphasizing foods that are strengthening, substantial, moistening, and lubricating. Vata types should avoid all gas-producing foods (cabbage, carbonated beverages) and stimulants (no more caffeine for you!). And Carolyn could not help but note that sour umeboshi plums are a power food for Vata types. The massage therapist was right!

Pitta: Fire

A Pitta, or Fire type, has a lot of things going for him (or her): courage, valor, good judgment, keen intellect, clear and strong speech. But some Pittas can take all that intense Fire and be too critical and sometimes belligerent. All of the weaknesses of a Pitta type are inflammatory. Remember that the Fire Element is the life blood, and many of the Pitta weaknesses show up when the chemicals of Pitta are transmitted through the bloodstream and exuded through the skin. Pittas may be prone to excess bleeding, bruising, skin disorders, fever, excess thirst, nausea, diarrhea, and vomiting. Pittas need a diet that is cool, slightly dry, and somewhat heavy. They do best with bland, mild-tasting foods and should avoid excess oil, sour tastes, salt, and pungent flavors.

Kapha: Water

A Kapha, or Air type, is about endurance, potency, constancy. A Kapha type can be very forgiving and compassionate and is almost always easy-going. However, this type often has a sedentary lifestyle and has to fight to keep weight off. Obesity and diabetes are the demons a Kapha may face. The constancy of a Kapha can mean that person is resistant to change—and takes a romantic breakup hard, hard, hard. The weaknesses of the Kapha tend to be congestive—respiratory infections, swelling, and obstructions such as tumors and cysts. A Kapha type needs foods that are light, dry, and warming and have pungent, bitter, and astringent tastes. These types need to eat less food and less frequently.

Guidelines for Ayurvedic Food Types

Vata (Air)	Pitta (Fire)	Kapha (Water)
Warming, grounding	Cool	Light, dry, warming
Strengthening, substantial	Slightly dry	Pungent, bitter, astringent flavors
Moistening, lubricating	Somewhat heavy	Less food less frequently
Spices, especially with sweet or heavy food	Bland, mild tastes	Avoid heavy, oily, or creamy foods
Dairy	Sweet, bitter, astringent flavors	Avoid sweets, salt, or sour tastes
Avoid gas-producing foods such as beans, cabbage, broccoli, and nightshade vegetables (tomatoes, eggplant, green bell peppers)	Avoid spicy, acidic foods	Increase spicy foods; they boost metabolism
Drink plenty of liquids	Avoid oil, salt, alcohol, red meat	Beverages in moderation; avoid all chilled beverages
Fruits moisten and harmonize Vata; minimize dried fruits	Emphasize fruits, vegetables, low-fat dairy; minimize sour fruits such as grapefruit, lemons, peaches, apricots, papayas	Avoid sweet and watery fruits; avoid fatty fruits such as avocados and coconut
Sweets in moderation		
Cooked vegetables		

Soul Soothers

You may already naturally have cultivated soul soothers in your life. Now that you are more mindful of the Elements, you can tap into the healing qualities of each one. Arlene, with a strong Air influence, has to remind herself to breathe deep when she is anxious. If she does this, she will relax; if not, only more anxiety comes in. Here are some soul soothers we thought of. There's space here so you can fill in some of your own.

Fire	Earth	Air	Water
Soaking up sunshine	Climb a mountain	Travel	A swim in the ocean
Sauna	Building a sandcastle	Reading, writing	Hot tub
Crackling fire	Garden	Deep breathing	Warm bath
Hot stone massage	Petting a dog or cat	Talking it out with a friend	A contemplation fountain
Salsa dancing	Walking barefoot	Aromatherapy	Watermelon
Fireworks	Sand and stone candlescape	Hang gliding, parasailing	Hydrotherapy, hydrating facial mask
Carryout from a Thai restaurant	Walk in the woods	Hot-air ballooning	Swimming with dolphins; listening to dolphin tapes
_____	_____	_____	_____
_____	_____	_____	_____
_____	_____	_____	_____

Using the Elements to optimize your health can be a whole lot of fun, too! Now that you know what makes you tick, you are on your way to becoming the resident expert for your health. You can use Astrology, Tarot, and Psychic Intuition to guide you in when to cultivate the warmth and inspiration of Fire, the practicality and sensuality of Earth, the power thinking of Air, or the sensitivity of Water. Remember that most people are not perfectly balanced with the Elements. This thing called life is a process—a beautiful one, at that.

chapter 4

Attracting the Well-Being You Know You Want

The Sun: The picture of health
Love thyself: What Astrology can reveal
Tarot and your self-esteem
Psychic Intuition and kinesiology
Body image: An ode to yourself
Jupiter, Saturn, and weight gain/loss
Belief-shattering: Tarot affirmations
Tarot touchstones: A visualization

Attracting wellness and inner contentment is as natural as soaking up the sun. When you take in the warmth and light that life has to offer, you radiate more positive energy, and your vitality increases. When you exercise regularly, your stamina and strength increase. You can exercise longer, so you enjoy it more and are faithful to your routine. When you eat healthful foods, you have more energy—not to mention freedom from the guilt factor. Small successes lay the foundation for more success. Do you believe you deserve to be your most healthful self? Are you a magnet for health? Or are you unconsciously pushing your vitality away? Some deep-seated beliefs and entrenched patterns may be diminishing your best chance at health. In this chapter, we use the Intuitive Arts of Astrology, Tarot, and Psychic Intuition to tap into recognizing what might be holding you back from your best self.

The Sun ☉: The Picture of Health

Through the ages, through many cultures, the image of the Sun ☉ as the source of vitality is a common theme. Ancient Egyptians worshipped the Sun god Ra. In Greek mythology, the path of the Sun across the sky was believed to be Apollo racing his chariot of fire. In Stone Age times, one of the first sciences was that of the sundial, measuring the length of the shadows caused by the Sun. In modern culture, there are Sun-worshippers, too, on the beaches of the world.

When you think of the Sun, you think of brightness, brilliance, warmth, light, nourishment. The Sun is the center of the solar system, and so it is the orientation point for Astrology. Your Sun ☉ sign symbolizes you as an individual—your spirit and your vitality. In Astrology, the Sun is the planet of light and growth. In Tarot, the Sun card is the archetype of happiness, contentment, and vitality for continued longevity.

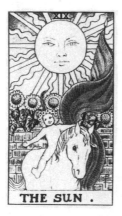

Tarot's Sun shines health and longevity upright. When reversed, the Sun could indicate a health challenge.

For that reason, the Sun card is the starting point in your journey of attracting the health and well-being you seek. This card represents one of the last steps on the journey of life. Take the Sun card out of your deck now and study the imagery. The dominant image is a bright, brilliant Sun. The child on the horse is innocent. His posture is open and nondefensive. He is unclothed, and he has nothing to hide. He is riding a strong horse—he has strong support and means to get where he is going. The four sunflowers represent a flourishing spirit. The billowing red cape represents free-spiritedness and contentment. Indeed, this card is all about contentment—contentment in marriage, in career, in all endeavors. It's a contentment that comes from within.

On the other hand, when the Sun card comes up reversed, it can point to what is holding you back from your best self. In essence, the light of the Sun is blocked. Your future is clouded, and your health is compromised. You are experiencing delays in understanding a life lesson. It may indicate that low self-esteem or childhood issues are blocking your development. When this card comes up reversed, obstacles are ahead, and you have not been equipped to meet your health challenges. It is a time to seek counsel and support.

Are you radiating positive health? Do you let your light shine? Good health begins with tapping into your natural radiance. The first step is to look at what is blocking the light and casting shadows in your life. Once you start removing the obstacles you have set before yourself, you will tap into a positive, powerful energy that can attract more and more vitality.

Do you love yourself? In her book *Revolution from Within,* Gloria Steinem (a pioneering Aries ♈) said, "I began to understand that self-esteem isn't everything; it's just that there's nothing without it." Nathaniel Branden, author of *How to Raise Your Self-Esteem* and other books, said, "Of all the judgments we pass in life, none is more important than the judgment we pass on ourselves." And maybe *I Love Lucy* star Lucille Ball (an ebullient Leo ♌—are you surprised?) said it most plainly: "I have an everyday religion that works for me. Love yourself first, and everything else falls into line. You really have to love yourself to get anything done in this world."

Self-esteem is the key to attracting your best, most healthful self. Do you take better care of your children or your career—or your car—than you do yourself? Your self-esteem is the foundation of all of your beliefs about your body, mind, and spirit and the way you deserve to be treated. If you are like most people, you probably love yourself in some areas of your life, but less in other areas. Do you believe your body works well? Do you believe in its innate healing power? Do you believe your body possesses the knowledge to nourish and replenish itself? Or do you see yourself as a collection of aches and pains—a wounded soldier on the losing side in the battle with time? Do you ever describe yourself as decrepit, falling apart, distracted, losing your mind, or rotting away? If so, we would like to show you how the Intuitive Arts can help you to be mindful of the language you use to refer to yourself.

In her book *You Can Heal Your Life,* Louise L. Hay says that when people come to her with a problem, whether it's poor health, money woes, an unfulfilled relationship, or stifled creativity, she works only on one front: guiding the person in self-love. Hay believes unloving thoughts create illness in the body. A Course in Miracles, a unique self-study spiritual thought system that teaches love and inner peace, says it this way: "All disease comes from a state of unforgiveness."

Hay offers this list of ways we don't love ourselves. Do any of them fit *you?*

- ☯ Self-criticism, scolding
- ☯ Mistreatment of the body with food, drugs, or alcohol
- ☯ A belief that you are not lovable
- ☯ A pattern of not asking for enough monetary compensation, either in charging for your services or seeking a job that pays well
- ☯ Creation of illness
- ☯ Creation of pain
- ☯ Procrastination in pursuing "bliss" agenda—the things that enrich your best self
- ☯ An environment of chaos, clutter, disorder
- ☯ Debts, burdens
- ☯ Attractions to lovers/mates who diminish or block you

Love Thyself: What Astrology's Houses Reveal

To get a glimpse into what your personal Astrology can tell you about your self-esteem, let's take a look in a few of the astrological houses. Remember, the 12 houses of Astrology represent the stages where you play out your life, and 4 of the houses represent your strongest health influences. They are called the angular houses. Think of the 1st house as your identity project. The 1st house rules your body, your health, your personality—essentially, your self. The 4th house defines your roots, your home, and your family. The 7th house rules your primary relationships—marriage and partnerships. The 10th house reveals your contribution to society through your career and community leadership. If your experiences in marriage, business, career, and community have been positive, your self-esteem will be higher.

Two other houses can give clues to your self-esteem. Because the 6th house is about service, health issues can show up there when you are giving too much in service to others and it is diminishing your health. If health has been a lifelong challenge for you, take a look at what's going on in your 12th house. This is the "karma" house, revealing deeply buried issues from your past. When health problems show up here, they always relate to long-standing patterns.

Let's take a look at the astrological birth chart of Britain's Princess Diana, who struggled with self-esteem even as she projected a joy and radiance to the world that still fascinates us many years after her untimely death. Remember that Diana suffered from bulimia, which she said was a response to her deeply unhappy marriage and her parents' divorce when she was a child. Diana's birth chart reveals that she was a Cancer Sun ♋ ☉ sign.

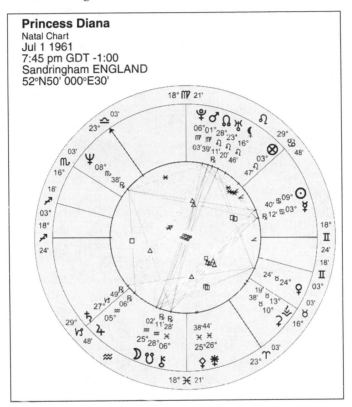

Princess Diana's birth chart.

Diana has Sagittarius ♐ rising in her 1st house, which represents body, personality, and public self. This is how we saw her: confident, enthusiastic, cordial, and happy to be with people. A Sagittarius ascendant has a good constitution and can recuperate from illness quickly.

To look at how Diana formed her self-esteem, we look at her 4th house, which reveals clues about her family of origin. That house is ruled by Aries ♈, which indicates a crisis in early childhood that would affect her most deeply. Mars ♂, the planet that rules Aries ♈, tells us that separation or early loss in the family dynamic cut to her core.

Looking at Diana's 7th house reveals a lot about her health, because it is the house of marriage, and we know her unhappy marriage caused her deep despair. She has her own natal Cancer Sun ♋ ☉ as well as natal Cancer Mercury ♋ ☿ in the 7th house. Both indicate Diana strongly identified herself in her marriage partner and the public, tending to want to nurture and be of service to them more than to her self. These planetary placements in the 7th house indicate that in a rocky marriage, she would take it on as if she were the one to blame. Mercury ☿ retrograde ℞ in that house points to many ups and downs for Diana as she tries to communicate her needs.

Diana's 10th house—the one of community leadership—has Neptune ♆ in Scorpio ♏, which points to Diana becoming a leader in an inspirational way. Neptune indicates her contributions to her world would not be forgotten, though she may not see herself in that way. Neptune always likes to keep a little mystery about it.

Diana's 6th house—service to others—is ruled by Gemini ♊, and the planet that rules Gemini—Mercury ☿—is next door in the 7th house. This indicates Diana would be very willing to help others, her partner, and the public to attain their goals. Mercury is the educator, and that would put education high on Diana's list, for herself and others. She studied health issues and sought to learn about maintaining a healthy mind, body, and spirit. Earlier in life, she gave too much of herself, but later in life, she became more conscious of her own health and spirit and shared that with the public.

Sagittarius ♐ is the sign in Diana's karmic 12th house and there are no planets in that house—what that tells us is that her karma was to personify the Sagittarius sign. As a duty to herself, she would need to become outgoing, not be afraid to say what's on her mind, to be self-actualized, not be a follower but a leader. Her karmic lessons would be to become more independent and self-reliant, and not to worry about what others thought or wanted her to become.

To that, Arlene says, "Bravo!" Diana certainly accomplished much of the task of building her confidence. She became able to speak the truth about herself and her marriage, and she developed herself as an inspirational Sagittarian communicator.

Health in Your Houses

What do Astrology's houses reveal about *your* health and well-being? Look in your birth chart and complete the following table, looking at the planet(s) and their sign(s) for your 1st, 4th, 7th, and 10th houses, and then for the supplemental influence of the 6th and 12th houses. Note if any of the planets are retrograde ℞, which could indicate a potential health blockage or lesson to be learned. (You'll find out more about retrogrades in Chapter 6.)

Astro House	Planet(s)	Astro Sign(s)	What It Means for Your Health
1st (body, health, personality)	_____	_____	_____
4th (roots, home, family)	_____	_____	_____
7th (marriage and partnerships)	_____	_____	_____
10th (contribution to society)	_____	_____	_____
6th (service to others)	_____	_____	_____
12th (karma and long-standing patterns)	_____	_____	_____

Your Self-Esteem: A Tarot Spread

Let's see what the Tarot has to tell you about your personal health opportunities and challenges. We use a Four-Card Spread here, with each card representing the four primary self-esteem houses—1st house of body and self, 4th house of family, 7th house of marriage and partnership, and 10th house of community leadership.

1st House
Body and Self

4th House
Family

7th House
Marriage and
Relationship

10th House
Community
Leadership

Self-Limiting Beliefs: Psychic Intuition and Kinesiology

Over time, we form beliefs about our bodies and what they can do—and not do—for us. For instance, if you struggle with allergies and asthma, you may have gotten the message early on that you could only expect so much from your body. If you are entering middle age and have always been blessed with endless energy—or if you just became a parent and are experiencing sleep deprivation for the first time (read: Carolyn, a healthy but sleep-deprived Sagittarius ♐)—you may be getting your first message about the limitations of your health. We form beliefs over time based on these messages. Sometimes we hold on to these beliefs long after we need them.

Self-limiting beliefs are deep-seated. One way to get to the root of your self-limiting beliefs about your body, mind, and spirit is through transformational kinesiology. Kinesiology is a holistic energy-balancing method, and it is based on the science of movement—quite literally, in Greek, the word *kinein* means "to move," and *logos* means "to study." By monitoring the energy required for a muscle to fire, a trained kinesiologist can collect biofeedback—information about the body—to identify self-limiting beliefs, stressors, and energy blockages.

One technique involves having you speak aloud a statement such as "I believe I am loved for who I am" three times. As you speak, you are instructed to push against the arm or hand of the practitioner. The practitioner is trained to identify whether the resistance is strong or weak. If you are skeptical about this, then think about it this way: If you were asked to say, "I believe I am beautiful and powerful," out loud to another human being who might judge you and might or might not support your belief, could you say it confidently? Say it out loud now, three times, and notice how you say it. Listen to the dynamics of your voice. Notice what thoughts go through your mind as you say it. Did doubts come up? Did your judgment side kick in, to discern whether it was true? Did thoughts come in of times in your life when you got the message that you weren't beautiful or powerful or loved for who you are?

These are the pointers to Psychic Intuition, the "I know but I don't know how I know" side of you. When you speak out loud a statement in the affirmative of something you don't truly believe about yourself, you will say it differently. Think of it as your body, mind, and spirit's way of telling the truth. You know when you don't believe with every cell of your being. It feels unnatural to say "I am strong" or "I have endurance." Thoughts immediately flood in to qualify the message, as in

"I am strong sometimes, but not other times." "I was strong when I was younger, but I'm not now."

Let's make a list of positive statements about your body, mind, and spirit, inspired by Tarot's Major Arcana. Try these statements, saying each out loud three times.

From the Fool: I believe I am safe.

From Temperance: I believe I am loved for who I am.

From Wheel of Fortune: I believe I can get my needs met.

From the Chariot, Strength: I believe I am a strong person.

From the High Priestess: I believe I can trust my inner voice.

From the Star: I believe I am beautiful, inside and out.

From the Empress: I believe I am graceful.

From the Magician: I believe I can accomplish anything.

From the Lovers: I believe I am attractive to the opposite sex.

From the Tower: I believe I am resilient.

How did that feel? Which ones felt right to you? Which ones didn't quite fit you—or so you believed? Make some notes right now in your Intuitive Arts notebook.

Body Image and Self-Talk

Remember from Chapter 1 that astrological signs rule certain body parts? Check which body part is ruled by your Sun ☉ sign and take the time now to celebrate the marvel of how it functions, how it looks, how it feels to touch it. How do you *really* relate to your body and its various parts—are you living in mind, body, spirit harmony?

Oprah Winfrey reaches many people because of her willingness to be open about her personal struggle with weight and body image; Oprah's birth chart appears in Chapter 3. This time, let's revisit Astrology's houses and look in Oprah's chart to see where her health challenges and opportunities are, and how she uses her experiences to help others.

Mercury ☿, the communicator, rules Virgo ♍, and we find Virgo on the cusp of Oprah's 1st house—the house that shapes the image she projects to the world. Oprah's 1st house shows us she feeds her self-esteem through her ability to get people to communicate about issues deeply felt and related to their personal growth. It shows us she would share her personal struggles with health with the public.

Oprah's Moon ☽ in mutable Sagittarius ♐ falls in her 4th house—and Oprah's 4th house is ruled by Jupiter ♃. This shows us that issues

79

from Oprah's family of origin held her back emotionally early in life, but she would need to speak the truth later in a way that healed herself and others. Oprah's 10th house, the house of community leadership, has talk-in-motion Gemini on the cusp and includes Jupiter ♃, the planet of good fortune and growth. This shows us her career would expand as she struck a chord with the public. Oprah's mercurial rulers show us that getting a genuine response from her audience is vital for her self-esteem and the way she measures her career accomplishments. Mercury ☿, the communicator, who shows up in Oprah's 6th house, the house of service, indeed relates Oprah's powerful ability to share her ideas, moving her audience to think about their lives. Mercury in Aquarius ♒ indicates a need to communicate on humanitarian issues. Because the fixed air sign of Aquarius is in her 6th house, it tells us quite a lot about the *way* she serves. It indicates great feeling for the human condition.

Mutable Pisces ♓ shows up in Oprah's 7th house, the house of partners. It indicates Oprah would relate compassionately to her public, but also she would need the public to empathize with her challenges. Pisces is famous for universal compassion—the ability to walk a mile in someone else's shoes—and Oprah certainly has done that!

Transformative Pluto ♇ in the fixed sign of Leo ♌ falls in Oprah's karmic 12th house—indicating she has a spiritual obligation to help others. She has an intense need to get others to understand they can transform their fears and triumph in the face of adversity. But she strongly needs the support and encouragement from her public to complete her karmic duties.

Jupiter ♃, Saturn ♄, and Weight Gain

While our goal here is that you love yourself, pounds on or pounds off, we do want you to know you can use Astrology as your weight-loss ally. Know that when jolly Jupiter ♃ passes through your Sun ☉ sign, you are more susceptible to weight gain. And when sober Saturn ♄ moves through your Sun sign, the pounds melt away effortlessly. In late 2003, the Sun signs prone to weight gain were Leo ♌ and Virgo ♍, but Leos were in for more of a struggle. That's because Leo likes to live on the largess of life. Leo goes for everything in a big way—and that means food, too—not just any food, but rich food. Leos have a sophisticated palate, and they love abundance. Virgos, on the other hand, tend to exercise more and gravitate to fresh fruits and vegetables. Saturn has a slimming effect when it passes through your Sun sign because it encourages practicality and discipline. Think of Saturn as a stern personal trainer.

To say that Jupiter is passing through your Sun sign is the same as a Jupiter transit, a term that you have probably encountered in daily astrological reports in the newspaper or on the radio. Transits are the "real time" movements of the planets through the signs, and affect everyone. That is, when Jupiter moves into Leo, it's in Leo for everyone. How much a transit affects *you* is determined by your birth chart. Think of planetary transits as actors entering the stage, about to speak and set new events in motion for your life. For instance, when either Jupiter or Saturn transit over your Sun sign or ascendant, sometimes even your 6th house, you may experience a dramatic change in your eating habits. Case in point: Here is Oprah's chart during a Jupiter transit, a time in her life when her weight proved a challenge.

An ephemeris of the daily planets can guide you in determining what planets are transiting through what signs at any given time.

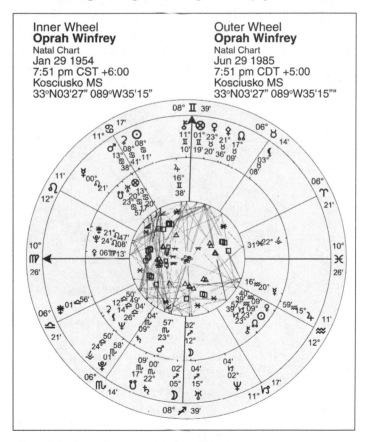

Oprah's chart during a Jupiter transit.

Belief-Shattering: The Role of Affirmations

In your self-talk about your body, do you talk in punishing terms, or are you compassionate and forgiving? Can you delight in the physical sensations of the body? Can you easily experience sexual pleasure? Do you have a balanced view of food? Or do you overindulge? Do you shame yourself when you let yourself indulge—even a little? Can you say you have a profound reverence for your body and its sacredness? Can you appreciate all of its functions? Can you love all of your imperfections? Can you delight in all of its quirks—from your bony knuckles to your gurgling stomach? (Notice we didn't ask you whether your spouse or partner can delight in your body's quirks. It's only necessary that *you* do.) Can you delight in all of its wonders—the miracle of how this collection of cells, with all of your thoughts, good and bad, all of your memories, all of your spirit, is uniquely *you?*

If you struggle with any of these, you may need to shatter some old beliefs about your body and replace them with new affirmations. Notice we have again borrowed some archetypes from the Tarot. We filled in some belief-shattering affirmations so you get the idea, but have left room for you to fill in your own.

Old Belief	New Belief and Affirmation
I'm tired all the time. I don't have any stamina.	**The Fool** I am enthusiastic about life and filled with energy for the people and activities I love.
I am weak. I must ask other people to help me with tasks that require muscle power.	**Strength, Queen of Swords** I am strong. I have the power and strength and knowledge to handle anything.
I'm just a klutz.	**Temperance** I am graceful and sure-footed.
I am fat.	**The Sun, 3 of Cups** I am protected and loved unconditionally. All that I need has been provided for me. I am well taken care of.
I can't rely on my body. I get sick so often and so easily.	**The World, 9 of Cups** All that I need has been provided for me. I have the power and strength and knowledge to handle anything.

Old Belief	**New Belief and Affirmation**
______________________	______________________
______________________	______________________
______________________	______________________
______________________	______________________
______________________	______________________

Health Challenges and Opportunities

Another way of looking at how you can use challenges and opportunities in your astrological birth chart to enhance health is to look at how the planets line up with each other—in other words, how they get along. These are called aspects, and they are determined by the planet's point on the birth circle, measured in degrees on a circle. (No, we won't make you do any geometry. We promise.) There are five major aspects.

- **Conjunctions ☌.** The strongest of the aspects.
- **Squares □.** Considered to be challenging. Their tension often yields dramatic action in your life. Degree: 90°
- **Oppositions ☍.** Like *yin* and *yang,* opposing planets show the need for balance between two competing energies. Degree: 180°
- **Trines △.** Considered the most favorable aspects. Their signs usually share the same Element: Air, Fire, Water, Earth. Degree: 120°
- **Sextiles ✶.** Considered harmonious. These bring about opportunities and attract possibilities. Degree: 60°

There are other aspects, too, but for now, we are going to concentrate on your challenges—squares □ and oppositions ☍, and opportunities—trines △, sextiles ✶, and conjunctions ☌. You can see the aspect symbols in the center of your birth chart wheel, showing how the planets aspect each other in the houses and signs. You can also see the aspects in a triangular aspect grid.

Let's take a look at the astrological birth chart and aspect grid of athlete Tiger Woods.

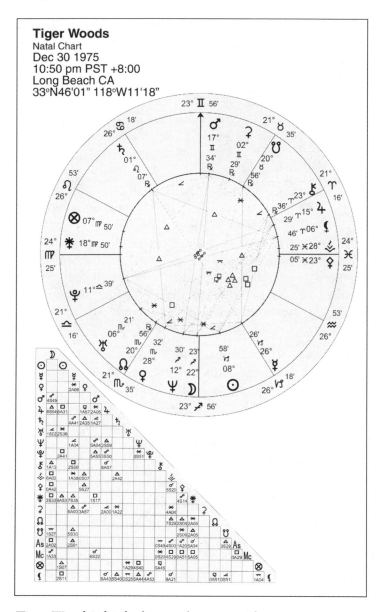

Tiger Woods's birth chart and aspect grid.

We will delve into aspects more in subsequent chapters, but let's take a quick glance at what Tiger's aspects might reveal. By looking at the number of favorable aspects—conjunctions, trines, and sextiles—

and challenging aspects—squares and oppositions—we can get the "exit poll" version of how his aspects influence his success. Tiger has an abundance of conjunctions, trines, and sextiles. Trines △, remember, are the most favorable aspects, while sextiles ✶ are those that bring opportunities. Certainly, winning the Masters at age 21 and then at age 25, holding all four major golf championships at once, Tiger is a man of opportunity. Trines easily outnumber all other aspects, making him a very lucky man, both in his talents and with the people who surround him. He knows what he wants and is blessed with personal drive and many supporters in accomplishing his goals.

Tiger has a surprising number of squares and oppositions that present challenges to him. These challenging aspects make him intent upon a goal, overcoming inner frustrations (squares □) and struggles with decision-making (oppositions ☍). They indicate he would develop a toughness, a unique ability for self-examination of imperfections and the ability to rise above them. Conflicts or defeats tend to fire him up and tap into his courage to change.

You can do a quick Headline News version of your aspects simply by counting them up using the triangular aspect grid that appears with your birth chart. As you do, certain patterns may immediately emerge. For instance, right away we can see that Tiger Woods has a lot going on with Jupiter ♃, the planet of expansiveness, opportunity, and pure good luck, and in Mercury ☿, the planet of communication. Take a few moments to make some notes about your aspect count from your birth chart. You may want to mark some of the planet-to-planet relationships that intrigue you so that you can come back to them later.

Tarot Touchstones: A Visualization

Visualization can be a powerful transformative technique. In this segment, we use Tarot to create a vision for the healthy person you want to be—and a road map for how to get there. This exercise involves five core questions that will help you shape your vision. First, shuffle the deck, and then divide it into three stacks. This is called "blessing" the deck. It represents the divinity of the mind, body, spirit union. Preparing the deck is an important ritual to use before asking some of your most heartfelt questions of the Tarot. For each question, choose a card and lay out the cards in a row, left to right.

Card 1: _____   Who is the person that is the
                                      healthiest me?

Card 2: _____   What does that healthy me do
                              for a living?
Card 3: _____   Where does that healthy me
                              live?
Card 4: _____   Who does that healthy me
                              love?
Card 5: _____   What does that healthy me eat?

Now, the picture of the healthiest you begins to come into focus. Let's use Tarot to create a road map to attract your best health. We will call these Tarot touchstones. You can use the Tarot to meditate on the touchstones each day. However, we don't want to leave you with a list of "shoulds." You probably have plenty of those in your head already. Know that real life is having one area of your life working well as you are challenged in another area. Use the Tarot touchstones to appreciate what is working, and make the decisions you need to make to enhance the other areas.

Tarot Touchstone 1: Nurturing Positive Relationships

To assess whether you have the kind of relationships depicted in the 10 of Cups—the relationships you need in your life to thrive—check whether these statements are true:

- ❏ I have a soulmate—many soulmates.
- ❏ I am close to my family of origin.
- ❏ I have built around myself a family of the heart.

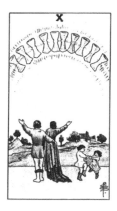

The 10 of Cups represents success in family, marriage, and love.

This touchstone is not so much about whether you are married in the happily-ever-after fairy-tale sense—it's more about whether you have surrounded yourself with intimate, affirming connections. A soulmate is someone to whom you are intimately connected—a connection that may transcend conventional boundaries of time, place, and legalities. It may be your spouse, but you may have other soulmates, too—a life-long friend you speak to once every few years, but still have a deep connection with, someone who supports your highest and best self. Can you say there is someone in your life that you can bare your soul with? Is there someone who knows most of your life events? Is there someone to whom you would feel comfortable confessing almost anything—and you know you would receive nonjudgmental compassion and wise counsel? This is known in psychology as the "nonblaming other" or "unconditional positive regard."

Ideally, you got this in your family of origin, but too many of us did not. The test here in this area is whether you have faced some of the issues that came up in your less-than-perfect family. Have you been able to take the love that was offered—and be at peace with the imperfect love that remains? Have you been able to create around you a family of the heart—people who are not your flesh and blood but who love you like family? You need both—a family of blood and a family of the heart. Sometimes your family of blood can only see you as a child or a younger sibling—as you were in your formative, less-evolved years—and can be blind to the person you have become. But sometimes your family of the heart doesn't have the history and deep ties—the unquestioning capacity to sacrifice on your behalf—you find with a family of blood. Cultivate both in your life.

We offer these principles as a test for creating a family of the heart, adapted loosely from Gloria Steinem's guidelines for a psychic family outlined in her book *Revolution from Within*:

- Can each person speak and feel heard?
- Does being part of this family of the heart make you feel more empowered? Does it challenge you to be your best self?
- Do you look forward to gathering with your family of the heart?
- Can you be honest? Can you be vulnerable? Can you trust the responses you get?
- Does being part of this family of the heart lead you to positive and independent action outside of it?
- Does the group honor the departure of old members and welcome new ones?

- ☾ Does being part of this group give you pride?
- ☾ Do you feel accepted as you are?
- ☾ Does the group make you stretch? Do you find you are becoming better than you thought you could be?
- ☾ Is there a balancing over time between what you're receiving and what you're giving to others?

Tarot Touchstone 2: Nurturing Positive Careers

If you work full time, then you work at least 40 hours a week. Consider there are only 168 hours in a week, and 56 of them are spent sleeping— at least, for those of us who get 8 hours of sleep each night. That means that of the 112 waking hours in a week, more than one third of them are spent at your job. That's why it's so important to your health that you thrive at work, the energy depicted in the 10 of Pentacles.

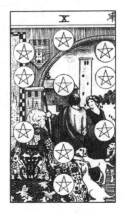

The 10 of Pentacles represents success in family, fortune, work, and material things.

To assess whether your work is enhancing or diminishing your health, check whether the following statements are true:

- ❏ My work is valuable to others.
- ❏ My bosses/clients value my work.
- ❏ My work contributes to my personal growth. I am always learning something new about myself.
- ❏ I have colleagues who inspire and support me.
- ❏ I feel energized at the end of the workday. I rarely feel drained.
- ❏ My ideas are valued, and my talents are used well in my work.

❏ My work contributes to a larger vision I have for my life.

❏ I have a mentor who guides and encourages me in my work.

Tarot Touchstone 3: Nurturing Personal Growth

How easy is it for you to grow and change? Do you have to be in a lot of pain, like the Hanged Man, before you are willing to let go? To assess where you are on the personal growth curve, check whether these statements are true:

❏ I can forgive easily.

❏ I can admit when I'm wrong.

❏ When I am in emotional pain, I want to know what I can learn from it.

❏ I am open to personal change.

❏ I am always seeking deeper self-knowledge.

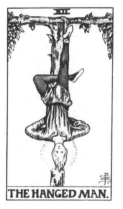

The Hanged Man represents releasing old patterns that cause pain.

Tarot Touchstone 4: Nurturing Your Home/Environment

How you care for your home is often a reflection of how you care for your body. If someone were to walk into your house, what would that person know about you? Would she see the flourishing home in the 4 of Wands? If you have a lot of photos of loved ones on the wall, she might conclude you care about your connections with others. If your walls are bare, she might conclude that you haven't really made your house a home.

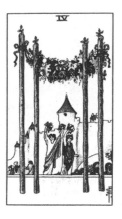

The 4 of Wands represents a flourishing home.

To assess this area, check whether these statements are true:

❑ I have a place in my home that I call my sanctuary. I can always go there to soothe my soul.

❑ My home is a place that expresses my sense of style.

❑ I think of home as a place where I can be myself and get my needs met.

❑ I love to create beauty all around me, in my home, at my desk, even in my car.

❑ I have a beautiful view from at least one window of my house (kitchen window, breakfast nook, picture window, courtyard or patio, sunroom).

❑ My bedroom is peaceful, a place of comfort.

Tarot Touchstone 5: Changing Your Energy

As we walk through these touchstones, you may see little areas that you want to change. You may see patterns emerging that you are now willing to let go of, now that you see the best person you can be and the new energy represented in the Death card. What does it take to change? This is where it gets harder. To assess where you are, check whether these statements are true:

❑ It's easy now for me to let go of negative relationships. I want to avoid negative people in my life.

❑ I have worked hard to heal my most hurtful relationships.

❑ I have gotten rid of all that stuff in my house that I don't need.

❏ I have a healthy outlet for anger and frustration.
❏ I know how to say no.
❏ I feel comfortable speaking my needs.

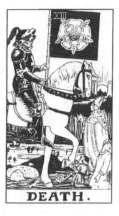

The Death card represents the power of changing your energy.

Tarot Touchstone 6: Radiating Positive Energy

Once you take the steps in touchstone 5, this one will flow naturally. It will seem effortless to radiate positive energy. The light represented in the Sun card, the card we began with at the start of this chapter, reflects the light within yourself today. The light shines well and bright, revealing a positive self-image, and attracts the good energy in people around you. Check whether these statements are true:

❏ I often compliment other people on the way they look or the way they responded in a certain situation.
❏ I show an interest in other people and their concerns.
❏ I believe that most people are honest and kind.
❏ I believe that most people are doing the best they can do at the time.
❏ I believe that all things work to the good.
❏ I believe I am loved for who I am.
❏ I believe in a power greater than myself, and I am connected to the universe, the Source, or the God of my understanding.
❏ I find it easy to discover simple joys in my daily life, even amid stressful situations.

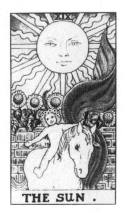

The Sun represents your most vital energy.

Health from Within

A healthy regimen is vital. But true health originates from within, from a deep love of self. From that can flow some of your best practices and experiences. It's about opening yourself up to the warmth of the Sun—and all that life has to offer.

chapter 5

Your Life in the Present Moment Is Beautiful, Too

The flow of life, the flow of you
True ease and calm abiding: Turn to the Tarot
Venus and Neptune: The "soft spots" in your astrological birth chart
From pain arises joy: Lessons from Tarot's Swords
The Dalai Lama: Direct your present to the future you desire
Beginner mind: The Fool
Wise innocence: The Hermit
Synastry: Healthy relationships

The teachings of Buddhism say the present moment is all that really exists. But if you are alive and breathing, you have no doubt had your share of trials with your health, whether it's the common cold, chronic pain, life's sorrows, or a major illness. Even if your health is not what you want it to be in the present, you can enjoy what is happening now. In this chapter, we use Astrology, Tarot, and Psychic Intuition to tap into some of the basic principles of Buddhism—calm abiding, mindfulness, compassion, being in the flow of life, acceptance. The ability to make friends with the present, even with all of its flaws, can equip you to advance, grow, and challenge yourself to the future health that you desire, and we show you how the Intuitive Arts can guide you.

Make Friends with the Present Moment

In her book *Joyful Mind*, Susan Piver describes meditation as the "noble act of making friends with yourself." But why is it so hard to stay *yourself,* true in the present moment? Astrology can help you get to know yourself, how you are constituted and how you approach life—and get comfortable with that, to say, "This is who I am." This knowledge can give you peace, love, and understanding about your past—a place to get clues about why you're headed the way you're headed. You can use the Intuitive Arts to keep past health problems and past fears and challenges from blocking your awareness of the beauty of the present moment, and to release the blossoming potential of the future.

Take time now to commit yourself to cultivating moments of peace in the present. Meditation allows us to sink into our own center—our body, mind, and spirit core. It can help us look at the ways we block our own awareness of peace. We do this when we say "Maybe I can have a better health routine after ... we move into the new house ... after I meet this deadline ...." Or "I can be happy after I get this job ... once I'm married ... if only I could have children ... once I lose 20 pounds ... after the surgery ...." This puts us in the position of always waiting, hoping, planning, never content in the right here, right now. Sometimes those times of transition—the journey to get to that place where we think happiness awaits us—*are* the happiest times. It is only when we look back, having arrived, that we realize a beautiful life unfolds in the process—and we know we must pay better attention.

Realize there will never be a day when all circumstances are "right"; yet each day can be a perfect day. Even as you look within a moment of loss or challenge, see the silver lining as well as acknowledge the grief or difficulty of the moment. Being happy in the moment despite external circumstances is the art of living—and the key to health.

Lunar Highs, Lunar Lows: Biorhythms of Life

To make friends with the present moment, we can use Astrology to gain insight into the rhythm of a day. In Chapter 2, we talked about how the Moon ☽ moving through the astrological signs can influence us, but did you also know the Moon phases have a pull on us? As the Moon tugs at the tide, it can tug at our energy. The Moon moves through four major phases in its 29½-day cycle. Understanding how everyone feels the pull of the Moon can help us work *with* the flow of life rather than *against* it.

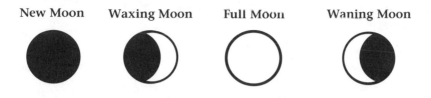

New Moon   **Waxing Moon**   **Full Moon**   **Waning Moon**

The Moon's darkest night—the Balsamic Moon—is a time just before it begins its next cycle. It is at this time that the energy of Psychic Intuition is at its peak. As part of the Last Quarter Moon, the Balsamic Moon represents closure to an old cycle or an end to old patterns in our lives.

Know also that you have a personal New Moon, which is called your lunar high. That occurs when the Moon ☽ is traveling through the same astrological sign as your Sun ☉ sign. Let's say you are a Gemini ♊, so you will feel your best when the Moon is dancing through Gemini. Your lunar low hits when the Moon is in the sign opposite your Sun sign. For a Gemini, that would be Sagittarius ♐. This is a time not to start any new health routines, because you will encounter obstacles.

Biorhythms study the natural rhythms of the human body, and one of the three primary cycles is tied to the Moon. The lunar cycle is your emotional biorhythmic cycle. The other two major biorhythmic cycles are the 23-day physical cycle and the 33-day intellectual cycle (your creative, problem-solving abilities). Some who study biorhythms add 3 more—a 38-day intuitional cycle, a 43-day aesthetic cycle (your interest in beauty and harmony), and a 53-day spiritual cycle (your inner peace, your openness to change). Biorhythms are the rise and fall of energies in each of these cycles. The cycles oscillate at regular intervals through your whole life.

It is easy to find out your biorhythmic cycle because there are many free calculators on the Internet, including www.1horoscope.com (which calculates all six), www.bio-chart.com, www.mybiorhythms.net, and www.facade.com/biorhythm. On the day Carolyn did her biorhythms, her physical and emotional cycles were at their lowest point, and her intellectual cycle didn't look good for several more days. She had had a winter cold for more than a week. Her sinuses ached, and a few days of decongestants put her brain in a haze. Carolyn's biorhythms called out for her to cultivate peace and calm abiding, to accept her energy as it was in the present moment and wait for a better day. Carolyn needed to acknowledge this as a time to be gentle and not expect so much of herself. Which, of course, brings us to the Tarot.

True Ease and Calm Abiding Through the Tarot

Many cards in Tarot's Major and Minor Arcana point to developing true ease with yourself or the situation at hand. Others point to calm abiding, a peace within—a time of trusting your intuition or celebrating the joy of life. Let's start with the Major Arcana. Lay them out once again in order, from the Fool to the World. Which four of these cards speak of ease with oneself? Which depict possessing deep intuition or seeking intuition? Make some notes about why you resonate to the cards you've chosen. Then go through the Minor Arcana and pick the four that are the most calming to you. Why?

When we did this exercise, these cards stood out: for the Major Arcana—High Priestess, the Hermit, Temperance, and the Moon. To that, we would add from the Minor Arcana the Queen of Cups, 4 of Cups, 4 of Swords, and 4 of Wands.

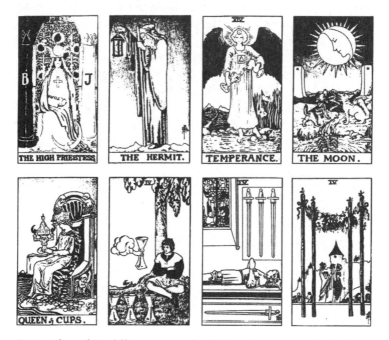

Principles of Buddhism meet the Major Arcana cards in the High Priestess, the Hermit, Temperance, and the Moon. In the Minor Arcana, we resonated to the Queen of Cups, 4 of Cups, 4 of Swords, and 4 of Wands.

Cultivating Your "Soft Spot": A Forty-Day Tarot Meditation

Use the Tarot to guide you to find your soft spot, the place where you can be vulnerable, from which kindness and forgiveness flow. When you find you can be soft with someone who previously would prompt you to put up your defenses, you will tap into a new wholeness. You are no longer in a struggle to protect yourself with a stressful fight or flight response. You can see a hurtful person or situation in the past with newfound compassion in the present—because you are whole.

It is uncanny how in many families a serious illness can unleash compassion that has been locked in a vault for decades. A threat to our health, or a loved one's health, often lifts us out of emotionally imprisoning and unforgiving thoughts. A parent or sibling we have held a grudge against for years suddenly seems vulnerable and human, just like us, when we witness that person's very real confrontation with mortality. Or, maybe the grudge you have is with yourself, and you haven't been kind to yourself.

All these questions can be asked of the Tarot to guide you to your soft spot, where the ice covering your heart starts to break into shards. Once you do, you can fully exist and be well. In Buddhism, this is called "metta," which literally means lovingkindness. It is the practice of generating compassion for all living beings, including oneself. This practice of lovingkindness, as illuminated by Buddhist guide Sharon Salzberg, involves meditating on the following:

May you be free from danger. May you be happy. May you be healthy. May you live with ease.

As you meditate, start with yourself and work your way to more difficult people. You start with yourself because, as the Buddha said, "You can search the entire universe for someone more deserving of your love and affection than you are yourself, but that person is not to be found anywhere. You, yourself, more than anybody in the universe, deserve your own love and affection." After yourself, you move to someone to whom you feel grateful, then to a beloved friend, to a neutral person, to someone with whom you have had conflict, and finally, to all beings everywhere.

To cultivate your soft spot, we recommend you try a 40-day daily Tarot meditation that can begin with the daily question to the Tarot, *"How can I be more compassionate to ...."* Fill in the blank with a name each day. The names can be different each day, or you may find one or two names keep coming up. You may find you have to stay on that person for 4 or 7 or 10 days in a row before it gets unstuck. You may find it uncanny that you get the Hanged Man 10 days in a row. The Hanged Man, the card of letting go and release, is a definite message. Remember, your own name should come up at least once in the 40 days.

Use Tarot's Three-Card Spread for this daily meditation to reveal your challenges and your strengths in extending compassion. Card 1 indicates you. Card 2 indicates the person you have selected: your partner for the day. Card 3 gives insight into healing yourself and your relationship. Take notes in your Intuitive Arts notebook each day and take the time to meditate on your soft spot, visualizing that place in your body from which forgiveness flows.

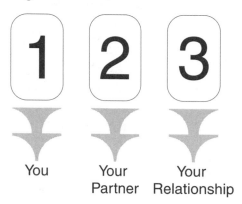

You   Your   Your
Partner   Relationship

Use this spread each day for 40 days to release compassion toward the people in your life, and heal your body, mind, and spirit.

Venus ♀ and Neptune ♆: The Soft Spots in Your Birth Chart

As we delve a little deeper into finding your soft spot, we focus on two planets in your astrological birth chart. Venus ♀ gives us insight into how we love, while dreamy Neptune ♆ gives us the ability to have compassion and forgive. Arlene, for instance, has Venus in Capricorn ♀ ♑, and the message for her is to receive her own love and not ignore it. Her Neptune is in Libra ♆ ♎, which means she can easily have compassion for others, but she needs to learn to forgive without needing a response in return.

Here are a few keywords for how Venus and Neptune through the astrological signs relate to the ability to be compassionate. Because Neptune moves so slowly—it hangs out in each sign for about 14 years—we have noted the birth years that fall under each sign. Note that the Neptune in Pisces ♆ ♓ folks haven't been born yet!

Venus ♀	How You Love	Neptune ♆	How You Forgive
In Aries ♈	Head over heels	In Aries ♈ b. 1862–1876 Inspires zeal and pioneering	First, foolishly sometimes.
In Taurus ♉	Take your time, can be possessive, strong aesthetic sense	In Taurus ♉ b. 1876–1890 Inspires through an aesthetic, industrious, materialistic approach	Through physical action. You often make up financially for any loss.
In Gemini ♊	Lighthearted, emotionally objective; commitment is hard, but you communicate well	In Gemini ♊ b. 1890–1901 Inspires through a perceptive, restless, inquiring approach	Through com- munication, in the written or spoken word.
In Cancer ♋	Romantic, sensitive, can be possessive, very nurturing	In Cancer ♋ b. 1901/02– 1914/16 Inspires through family	Through nurturing others' dreams and goals.
In Leo ♌	Flair for dramatic, generous, selfless, ardent	In Leo ♌ b. 1914/16– 1928/29 Inspires through entertainment, drama, and love	Need to overcome pride and ego. Just apologize.
In Virgo ♍	Sincerely affec- tionate, loves to serve others, discerning in love matters	In Virgo ♍ b. 1928/29– 1942/43 Inspires through public service	Through serving others.

Venus ♀	How You Love	Neptune ♆	How You Forgive
In Libra ♎	An uncanny creative knack for creating harmony and beauty, gracious, appreciative	In Libra ♎ b. 1942/43–1955/57 Inspires through beauty, art, music, idealism	Need to forgive indiscretions, failings in partnerships.
In Scorpio ♏	All-consuming passion, powerful	In Scorpio ♏ b. 1955/57–1970 Inspires through transformation, loss	Transcend old expectations of others; may hold grudges.
In Sagittarius ♐	Lighthearted, idealistic, adventurous, loves freedom, expansive	In Sagittarius ♐ b. 1970–1984 Inspires through spiritual practice and global interest	Educate and inspire others to find their individual truth; quick, blunt, and optimistic.
In Capricorn ♑	Careful, cautious, cautious, loyal, dedicated	In Capricorn ♑ b. 1984–1998 Inspires through Traditional conscientious leadership	Through others' despair, having compassion, observing their loss.
In Aquarius ♒	Can seem emotionally detached, cares about freedom and openness	In Aquarius ♒ b. 1998–2012 Inspires through altruism	Transcendent to a higher level of consciousness; allows for individual freedoms.
In Pisces ♓	Sympathetic, compassionate, can love too much, an unconditional love	In Pisces ♓ b. 2012–2025/26 Inspires through sacrifice, devotion and universal love	Through allowing and acknowledging the soul's evolution. Possess a healthful respect for personal transcendence.

The Dalai Lama says that compassion is what makes our lives meaningful. "It is the source of all lasting happiness and joy," he writes in *Ethics for the New Millennium: His Holiness the Dalai Lama* (Riverhead Books, 1999). "And it is the foundation of a good heart, the heart of one who acts out of a desire to help others. Through kindness, through affection, through honesty, through truth and justice toward all others we ensure our own benefit."

From Pain Arises Joy: Lessons from the Tarot Suit of Swords

Being mindful means being conscious of your body, mind, and spirit in the present moment. Being at peace with what that present moment holds is easier said than done. What if your day brings suffering? The temptation to dwell in the sweet memories of the past or dream of a better future is great when you are in immediate pain, whether the source is physical or emotional.

How can you transcend the pain of the present to find the peace? Begin by understanding pain's role in calling you back to health. Pain can be a signal to your body to stop, as in "Stop touching that hot stove!" It can signal where you have trapped energy that needs to be released through massage, exercise, or emotional catharsis. But pain can also be evidence of your body at work, as in childbirth. Each contraction is accomplishing the task of delivering a baby, moving it through the birth canal. When Carolyn was pregnant with the twins, she took a natural childbirth class from Pam England, author of *Birthing from Within*, who is a Zen Buddhist. England asked participants to visualize each contraction as moving the baby closer to the light, moving out of darkness. She asked participants to embrace the pain of each contraction, welcoming it to do its work, visualizing as each contraction approached its peak that this one was going to do a lot of work.

This is the opposite of our natural reaction to pain and suffering. Ask any woman who has ever experienced childbirth if when she was in labor, she felt welcoming and charitable to each contraction! But Zen master Thich Nhat Hanh, a Vietnamese Buddhist monk who is part mystic, part scholar, and part activist, says this of suffering, "When you understand suffering, a kind of energy is born in you, the energy of compassion, the energy of lovingkindness." That energy is healing energy. Pema Chodron is among the first group of Western women to be ordained as a Tibetan nun. In her book *The Places That Scare You*, she says at the core of our more painful experiences lie the seeds of spiritual awakening.

Let's take a look at what the Swords in the Tarot can reveal about the role of pain in awakening you to your best opportunity for health.

101

While the royal court of Swords represents balanced judgment and wise counsel before taking decisive action, the everyday cards of the Swords are about facing and dealing with life's conflicts. By taking a closer look at these cards, you can gain insight in your approach to pain and conflict. Once you develop a more thorough understanding of their meanings, you will be able to make your Tarot readings more effective. So get out your Tarot deck and sort out the Ace through 10 of Swords.

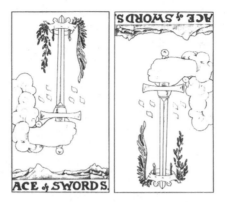

Ace of Swords. Keywords: Initiation, focus.

When the Ace of Swords appears, it reveals a new endeavor to be launched, and that it will prove to be victorious. This card speaks to you of your power. You may have just emerged from a difficult time with your health, but you are now tapping into your power and you are in control.

When the Ace of Swords is reversed, the sword is cutting to inflict pain. You are being warned that you are applying too much force to a situation about your health.

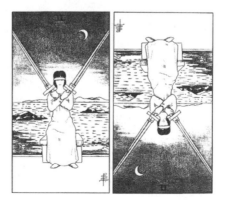

2 of Swords. Keywords: Blindness, emotional uncertainty.

The woman on the 2 of Swords card is blindfolded before the sea of her emotions, balancing two swords. The New Moon reveals she is at a moment of initiation, but blindfolded she cannot navigate her emotions to make a choice and take action. When the 2 of Swords comes up in the context of your health, you may be facing indecision. You may have inadequate information, or you may have received conflicting opinions from your doctors—or a recommendation from your doctor that conflicts with your own inner wisdom about your body. You must seek more guidance. When this card appears reversed, a decision has been made and action will be taken.

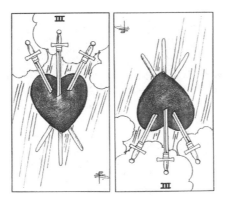

3 of Swords. Keywords: Sorrow, heartbreak.

Swords pierce the heart. Sorrow clouds the sky. The 3 of Swords can symbolize deep grieving, or it can indicate a separation. It may indicate a sorrow for loss of self—the person you once were in a happier, healthier time, or you as an innocent child. When it comes up in reading, the other cards around the 3 of Swords give context to the source of the sadness. This card implores you to get in touch with that sorrow and let the tears fall. It is the first step of compassion. When the 3 of Swords is reversed, it means you are working through a difficult heartache and setting the stage for healing and a new wholehearted future.

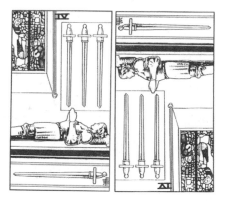

4 of Swords. Keywords: Rest, regroup, rejuvenate.

This card can signal a time to renew your energies, to rest comfortably. It can reassure you that it is the time for peace and you can rest in that calmness. It may be time for a vacation or retreat. If you have just had surgery or a round of medical care, it is a time of restoration and rejuvenation. When the 4 of Swords card is reversed, you are ready to get back in action on your health.

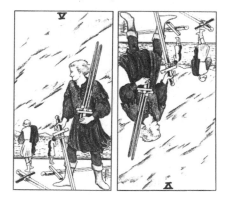

5 of Swords. Keyword: Selfishness.

The 5 of Swords shows insensitivity. The young man grips the swords with tenacious selfishness—"it's all about me." This card is about the misuse of power—vengefulness or destruction. In a reading, this card points strongly to the need for compassion and empathy to others. The cards around it point to why you have had difficulty summoning sensitivity and reveal the path to take to challenge yourself to move past it. When reversed, this card shows you are more aware of the need for compassion, but also reveals there is still some sneaky behavior and desire to create conflict.

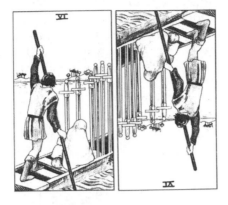

6 of Swords. Keywords: Release, calm, hope for the future.

In the story of the 6 of Swords, the sorrowful woman and her child are nearly imprisoned by the swords, which build a wall of separation between rough and calm waters as the ferryman pushes the little boat toward safe harbor. This card invites you to set sail toward tranquility. You will find that once you reach the opposite shore you have attained a higher state of consciousness and you can be at peace with yourself. You are healing. When this card is reversed, your journey to calmer waters is on hold.

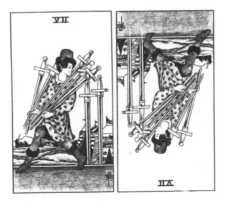

7 of Swords. Keywords: Deception, false information.

When this card appears, someone around you is unreliable, not trustworthy, deceiving you. Someone is threatening to steal from you that which you hold sacred. In the context of your physical health, this card in its most literal meaning can signal the need to ask the hard questions of your doctor or your insurance company. It is a time to be discerning about the information you are receiving, to test it against other sources. This card signals that it's time to ask "Is there another answer here?" In the context of your spiritual health, the 7 of Swords can point to someone in your life who you are allowing to diminish your health by letting that person violate your trust. Someone is stealing your energy. The other cards that come in the reading around it can point to who is hurting you and how to approach the situation. When this card is reversed in a reading, the deception is revealed, danger averted, and you are able to find a true and beneficial solution.

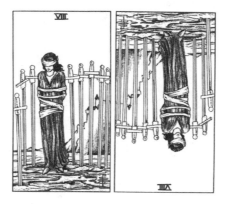

8 of Swords. Keywords: Fear, restriction.

This card reminds us that our fears can render us helpless and sightless. Fear has robbed this woman of her vision; sanctuary is so close but yet so far! When this card comes up, it's telling you that your course of action is limited. You have bound and gagged yourself—waiting for a sign! The woman may be too weak to fight for her rights, pinned down in a cycle of worry that leaves her blinded and unable to work for her own benefit. When this card is reversed, you have reached a point where you can let go of your fear and move toward the sanctuary of clear thought and well-being.

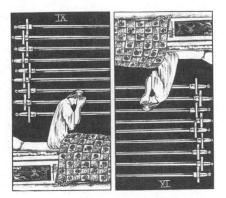

9 of Swords. Keywords: Despair, panic.

The woman in the 9 of Swords is paralyzed by pain, despair, plagued by nightmares and haunted by fears and worries about her situation. When this card comes up in a reading, the surrounding cards provide context about the source of the pain (whether it is physical, emotional, or spiritual), how quickly it will pass, and clues to resolving it. When the 9 of Swords is reversed, healing begins.

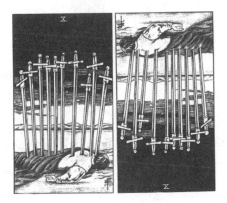

10 of Swords. Keywords: Catharsis, karmic completion.

Another ouch! The 10 of Swords depicts how a major trauma with our health can leave us feeling: It can wear us down and leave us feeling depleted and pinned to the ground. But this card reveals the end of a cycle. The source of the trauma has done its worst, the threat has subsided. When the 10 of Swords appears reversed, healing begins—perhaps even on a karmic level—signaling the beginning of a new and beneficial reality. Everything is new now, and the old conditions no longer apply as the swords fall away and you rise to walk toward a new dawn for your health and well-being.

Direct Your Present to the Future Health You Desire

The Dalai Lama tells us we can create our future potential, even from the pain of our present reality. Let's turn to the Tarot now and do a Diamond Spread. For this spread, Arlene posed the question, *"What is the future potential of my health?"* The four cards are read as a total essence of who you are now. Remember, you are the diamond at the center of the lotus blossom!

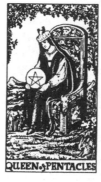
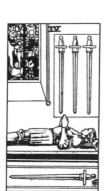
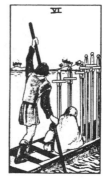
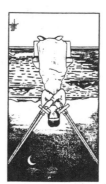

Arlene's Diamond Spread.

Let's look at the keywords for the cards of Arlene's Diamond Spread:

Card 1: 4 of Swords = rest and rejuvenation

Card 2: Queen of Pentacles = abundance, productivity

Card 3: 6 of Swords = release, calm, optimism

Card 4: 2 of Swords R = a decision has been made

What's your interpretation?

_____

_____

Beginner Mind Cultivates Wise Innocence

How can we create that beginner mind, a mind empty of self-imposed limitations? For that question, we turn to Tarot's Fool, the first card of the Major Arcana. In her book *Women Who Run with the Wolves*, Clarissa Pinkola Estes writes of cultivating a "wise innocence." Her book uses fairy tales and folk tales to illustrate psychological truths and insights. Wise innocence is about having walked the Tarot's archetypal journey of life, learning our lessons of temptation and regeneration, fortitude and compassion, we return to the beginner mind of Tarot's Fool—but now we are wiser. Innocence doesn't have to be foolish. Wise innocence lives in Tarot's Hermit.

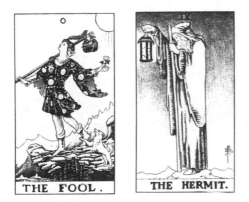

Tarot's Fool represents the beginner mind, and the Hermit, wise innocence.

In this exercise, we use Psychic Intuition and a meditation with the Hermit card from the Major Arcana. When Carolyn first got the Hermit card in a reading, she reacted with, "Oh no!" because she thought it indicated loneliness. But the Hermit is about seeking our inner truth.

The archetype that the Hermit represents is, indeed, the Dalai Lama. In the imagery of this card, the Hermit stands alone, high on a snowy (Tibetan?) peak, waiting and watching for others who come along the path. He holds the Lantern of Truth. The Hermit invites us to follow our own life path, resonating each step to our own unique and beautiful inner truth. But the Hermit also asks us to return to the beginner mind, the place of initiation and openness.

Take some time now to meditate on these concepts. What is holding you back from innocence? What has made you wiser?

1. Visualize yourself walking the path of Tarot's Fool, open and unprotected, your burden light. See yourself in the laughter and gaiety of youth, believing you will live forever and no accidents will befall you. There is no cliff.

2. Now sink deeper into yourself, visualizing that part of you where deep wisdom has collected. Sink into that for a moment, and honor it. Breathe deeply, directing your breath there. Place your hand on your belly as the breath fills your body. As you reach the peak of each inhalation, hold it there for one count before releasing it. Breathe through this six times as you connect with your deeper wisdom. Let the calmness wash over you.

3. Now see the armor around your heart that you have erected, as you have learned the lesson that others will try to harm you. Visualize that armor melting away, focusing now on your exhalations. See yourself seeing with new eyes—a night vision that sees into the distance, sees what others cannot see. See yourself illuminating your life path, holding up the Lantern of Truth to light the way for your innocent self to step forward to meet your wise self.

Accepting the Challenge: Astrology's Qualities

In this chapter, we talk about making peace with the present. But within that peace lives the challenge to advance, grow, change, and evolve. A deeper peace can come from embracing that challenge and feeling empowered to change.

Before we move on to how to use the Intuitive Arts to guide you in that change, however, let's take a look at how you are equipped to change. First, know that each astrological sign possesses a quality that defines your flexibility and adaptability. The qualities represent each season as it moves through its paces—a distinct beginning; a content, stable middle; and a transitional ending.

Astro Signs and Their Qualities

Cardinal	Fixed	Mutable
Aries ♈	Taurus ♉	Gemini ♊
Cancer ♋	Leo ♌	Virgo ♍
Libra ♎	Scorpio ♏	Sagittarius ♐
Capricorn ♑	Aquarius ♒	Pisces ♓

Cardinal. Independent—they are first of their season! If you are a Cardinal Sun ☉ sign, your strength will be in starting a new health regimen—exercise, meditation, or a better diet—and your challenge will be maintaining your interest in the middle of it. You are the type of person who needs to change your routine, adding new practices.

Fixed. Grounded—they are always where you can find them! The Fixed signs are the heart of the season, when summer's here or winter seems here to stay. If you are a Fixed sign, you are likely resistant to change. You may get stuck in a groove with your health habits, and it may be difficult to jolt yourself into a new routine or new awareness of self. You may need to place the other qualities, Cardinal and Mutable, around you to inspire you.

Mutable. Fluid—they are always in motion! One season flows into another—one day it's spring, the next it's winter again. Think of March, coming in like a lion and leaving like a lamb. Some days are gentle; some are fierce. Mutable signs thrive on this paradox, and do not find it unsettling in the least. You have the knack for seeing an issue from more than one angle. However, you may lack perseverance in sticking with a health regimen or a meditation discipline. You want to see the change. You may want to hook up with a Fixed sign as an encourager.

Carolyn is a Sagittarius ♐ with a Virgo ♍ rising, two Mutable signs, and she has found one of her favorite times of year is September through October, when those first crisp, cool days are interspersed with the golden yellow sun of Indian summer. Likewise, her favorite time of day is dusk, just before the day falls into night. If you are a Mutable Sun ☉ sign—it's intensified if you have another Mutable sign in your astrological power points—you are flexible, resourceful, and quick to learn.

The Synastry of Healthful Relationships

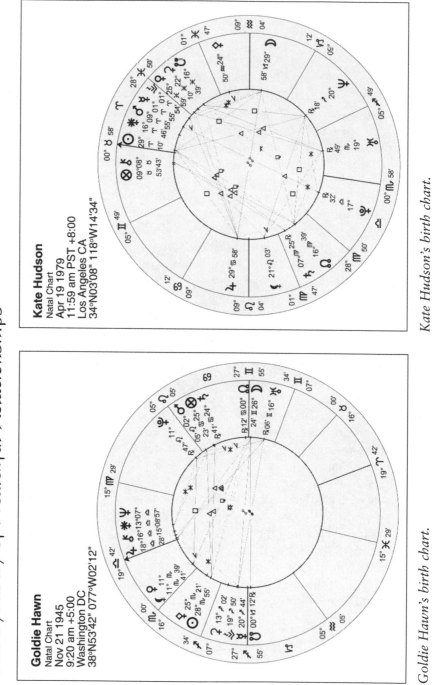

Kate Hudson
Natal Chart
Apr 19 1979
11:59 am PST +8:00
Los Angeles CA
34°N03'08" 118°W14'34"

Goldie Hawn
Natal Chart
Nov 21 1945
9:20 am +5:00
Washington DC
38°N53'42" 077°W02'12"

Kate Hudson's birth chart.

Goldie Hawn's birth chart.

Across
Goldie Hawn
Natal Chart
Nov 21 1945
9:20 am +5:00
Washington DC
38°N53'42" 077°W02'12"

Down
Kate Hudson
Natal Chart
Apr 19 1979
11:59 am PST +8:00
Los Angeles CA
34°N03'08" 118°W14'34"

	☽	☉	☿	♀	♂	♃	♄	♅	♆	♇	⚷	⚳	⚴	⚵	⚶	☊	☋	As	Mc	⊗	⚸
☽		⚹ 1S03			☍ 2A07		☍ 5S17	⚼ 1A08	△ 7A58				⚹ 4S38		∠ 1S56	⚻ 0A14				☍ 4S35	
☉	⚹ 2S45	⚻ 0S14	△ 8S26		□ 2A56		□ 4S28	∠ 1A56				△ 9S20			⚼ 1S07	⚹ 1A02	△ 1A02	△ 1S15		□ 3S46	
☿	□ 5S31	△ 3S00			△ 0A10		△ 7S14		☍ 6A01				△ 6S35			□ 1S43	□ 1S43	□ 4S01		△ 6S32	
♀	□ 0A25	△ 2A56		⚼ 0A39	△ 6A06		△ 1S18			⚼ 0A48			△ 0S39			□ 4A13	□ 4A13	□ 1A55		△ 0S36	⚼ 0A42
♂				⚻ 1A44	△ 7S49				☍ 1S58	△ 1A53	☍ 6A20		⚼ 0A26	☍ 3A13	△ 3A08						⚻ 1A47
♃		△ 1S02			☌ 2A08		☌ 5S16	∠ 1A08					△ 4S37				⚻ 0A15			☌ 4S34	
♄																	△ 7A13				
♅				☌ 8A11			△ 4S52						☌ 5S31							△ 5S34	☌ 8A08
♆	☍ 6S07		☌ 0S26			⚹ 1A50		☍ 4A12			⚹ 4A03	☌ 0A28			☌ 7A15				⚹ 0A36		
♇	△ 8S53					☌ 0S56		△ 1A26		⚹ 5A44	☌ 1A17	⚹ 2S18		☌ 4A24	⚹ 4A29				☌ 2S10		
⚷	∠ 2A42			☍ 2A56					⚻ 0S46	□ 3A05											☍ 2A59
⚳	□ 5S30	△ 2S59			△ 0A11		△ 7S13		☍ 6A02				△ 6S34			□ 1S42	□ 1S42	□ 4S00		△ 6S31	
⚴	△ 1A34	□ 4A05				△ 6S23	⚻ 0S09						□ 0A30			△ 5A22	⚹ 5A22	⚹ 3A04	△ 5S08	⚻ 0A33	
⚵			△ 3A57			☍ 1A42		⚹ 0S40		△ 4S59	☍ 0S31	△ 3A03		☍ 3S39	△ 3S44				☍ 2A56		
⚶	□ 4A14	△ 6A45	□ 1S26				△ 2A31					□ 2S20	△ 3A11					□ 5A44		△ 3A13	
☊			□ 4A05		∠ 0A27			□ 0S33				□ 3A11			□ 3S36						
☋			□ 4A05	△ 5S00	⚼ 0A27	⚻ 1A49		□ 0S33			⚻ 0S23	□ 3A11			□ 3S36						△ 4S57
As	∠ 2A20			□ 2A34	☌ 6A59				⚹ 1A08	☌ 2A43				⚹ 4A03	△ 3A58						□ 2A37
Mc	⚹ 4A34	⚻ 2A02			□ 1A08			∠ 0A08								⚹ 0A46	△ 0A46	△ 3A03		□ 5A34	
⊗	∠ 1A31			☍ 1A46					⚻ 1A56	□ 1A55											☍ 1A49
⚸	⚹ 5A22		△ 0S19			⚹ 2S35			∠ 1A54			△ 1S13	□ 4A18					△ 6A52	⚹ 1S21		

Goldie Hawn reads across and daughter Kate Hudson down on this astrological synastry grid.

So far, we have talked a lot about the influence of your personal relationships on your health. To get a better picture of how to analyze your astrological chart for ways that your relationships affect your health, we'll use Astrology's synastry to reveal healthful patterns for a famous mother and daughter pair, Goldie Hawn and Kate Hudson. Synastry is the Astrology of relationships. When using synastry, astrologers like Arlene look at how two birth charts relate to each other. Note that Kate's is a noon birth chart.

First, let's compare the basics:

Planets	Goldie's Astro Sign	Kate's Astro Sign
Sun ☉	Scorpio ♏	Aries ♈
Moon ☽	Gemini ♊	Capricorn ♑
Ascendant	Sagittarius ♐	Leo ♌
Mercury ☿	Sagittarius ♐	Aries ♈
Venus ♀	Scorpio ♏	Pisces ♓
Mars ♂	Leo ♌	Aries ♈
Jupiter ♃	Libra ♎	Cancer ♋
Saturn ♄	Cancer ♋	Virgo ♍
Uranus ♅	Gemini ♊	Scorpio ♏
Neptune ♆	Libra ♎	Sagittarius ♐
Pluto ♇	Leo ♌	Libra ♎

With Goldie's Sun ☉ in Scorpio ♏ and Kate's in Aries ♈, this is a powerful pairing, potent because of its varying energy. With ascendants in Sagittarius ♐ (Goldie) and Leo ♌ (Kate), two extroverted, exuberant signs, they may at face value seem very similar, but Goldie's Sun is in a Fixed Water sign—more tuned in to life's undercurrents—while Kate's Sun is in a self-starting, fiery, Cardinal sign. They definitely have different ways of approaching the world. These differences are challenging but constructive, and when we look closer at a synastry grid, we will see why.

In this synastry grid, read across for Goldie Hawn, down for Kate Hudson. Basically, a synastry grid looks at how the position of one planet in your chart relates to another planet in someone else's chart—whether it is opposite ☍, square □, trine △, sextile ✶, etc. A synastry grid is a readout of all of those aspects.

Goldie's Sun ☉ in Scorpio ♏ makes a sextile ✶ to Kate's Moon ☽, a well-grounded Capricorn ♑. It also trines △ Kate's Mercury ☿, Venus ♀, and Jupiter ♃. Goldie's Mars ♂ is making an aspect to every one of Kate's personal planets: Sun ☉, Moon ☽, Mercury ☿, Venus ♀, Mars, ♂, and ascendant. These strong aspects make this pair bonded from the start—lifelong partners and friends as well as mother and daughter. They play many roles together—Goldie as cheerleader, motivator, and "sister."

Saturn ♄, the planet of discipline and enduring lessons, has strong influences from Goldie to Kate. Saturn from Goldie's chart is a teacher to Kate in lessons that will last a lifetime, while Kate's Jupiter ♃ is sending generous, uplifting, lighthearted energy to her mother through its strong ties to Goldie's Sun ☉, Mars ♂, and Saturn ♄.

Remember, though, that our capacity for compassion and forgiveness is revealed in Venus ♀ and Neptune ♆, so let's focus there. Goldie's Venus is in Scorpio ♏, which shows her capacity for love and compassion is all-consuming, while Kate's Venus is in Pisces ♓, which indicates her compassion is intuitive and often unconditional and pure. Both of these indicate an innate ability to love and forgive; however, Kate's Pisces Venus ♓ ♀ is square ☐ to Goldie's Gemini Moon ♊ ☽, which may indicate that Goldie's way of talking through emotions may have been perplexing to Kate's intuitive nature at first. Kate's Neptune in Sagittarius ♐ is in opposition ☍ to Goldie's Moon ☽, but Goldie's Neptune trines △ Kate's Moon. This indicates Goldie, as the mother, may have led the way in forgiveness in their relationship, drawing upon the Neptune in Libra ♎ ability to see past small failings and indiscretions to the true beauty in a person—as mothers often do.

Now we invite you to get the birth chart for a significant person in your life and use Astrology's synastry to compare your two birth charts. Look to see how the charts reveal the ways in which health and well-being are encouraged or challenged by your relationship.

Take Me to the River

Now that you have begun to cultivate true ease and compassion, as you are also working to heal and foster beneficial relationships, a future healthier you can only flow from that wellspring. Think of your calm present as your gift to your future.

chapter 6

Been Down So Long, It Feels Like Up to Me

See your energy
Chakra check-in: Tarot and your life energy
War and peace: Mars in your astrological birth chart
Retrogrades: Health challenges and healing opportunities
The Jupiter track: Healthy optimism
The hope card: Tarot's Star
Healing bliss

Life's school of hard knocks can make us feel like Stallone's Rocky—down for the count. You may suffer from chronic health problems, or you may lack energy or feel blue most of the time. If you suffer from depression, if you're battling a chronic condition or illness, if you're trying to shed the pounds that bring health problems like diabetes or heart trouble, or if you have hit the wall with fertility treatments that already have left you battered and bruised, you may feel you have very little stamina left in you. How can you restore your hope? How can you keep moving, when what you'd really like is a 15-minute vacation from your own body? In this chapter, we help you identify and deal with personal health issues and longtime behaviors that may be holding you back from realizing your best well-being. We help you use Astrology, Tarot, and Psychic Intuition to get to the root of the problem and tap into your reservoir of fortitude. We help you effect positive internal changes that can set you firmly back on the path toward vitality.

So What's the Problem Anyway?

In this Psychic Intuition exercise, we help you step outside of your current health problems, see your energy, and redirect it. You need a partner—someone you know fairly well. Ask your partner to lie comfortably, someplace where you can sit at his or her head, with your fingers gently touching your partner's temples. You are barely making contact, lightly brushing your partner's skin with your fingertips—or not quite touching, just receiving this person's energy. Close your eyes and visualize the person's energy emanating up from the body into your hands.

As you do this, breathe deeply, gradually clearing your mind and focusing on your partner's health and well-being. Meditate on the many ways you know your partner, about the many roles she or he plays in life. Picture this person in different situations. Think about what your first impression might be if you met your partner now. After 10 minutes, consciously direct thoughts of healing and ease to your partner as you lightly press your ring finger into the spot between your partner's eyes—the third eye. The ring finger is ruled by the Sun ☉ and sends a warm energy of good will to connect and open understanding between you and your partner.

Below is a list of keywords we compiled to describe a person's energy. When you have completed the preceding exercise, consider what you have experienced of your partner's energy and check off as many as apply to describe your partner. Add others that occur to you.

Accepting	Expanding
Blaming	Falling
Blossoming	Fighting
Boiling	Fleeing
Burning	Flowing
Careering	Gathering
Caressing	Giving
Churning	Glowing
Clutching	Hardening
Contracting	Hiding
Criticizing	Laughing
Defending	Leaning
Denying	Longing
Draining	Opening
Drowning	Pinching
Escaping	Punishing

Radiating
Rebelling
Receiving
Refusing
Rejecting
Releasing
Resisting
Restricting
Retaining
Rising
Running
Shaming
Shrinking
Smothering
Soaring
Softening
Starving
Stewing

Stopping
Straining
Struggling
Supporting
Taking
Tempting
Tensing
Trusting
Tugging
Unaccepting
Wavering
Withholding

_____

_____

_____

For the next part of this exercise, you switch roles. You are lying down with your eyes closed, and your partner kneels or sits at your head, tuning in to *your* energy. As you participate in this part, do your deep breathing, tuning in to your own energy.

Finally, take a few minutes together to explore what kind of dis"ease" or malady might have its root in the energies you and your partner identified for each other. We've listed some associations here, but remember this exercise is intuitive and its aim is to activate your Psychic Intuition so that you can see clearly how it can be an ally to you in tending to your health. This is a version of the process used by gifted medical intuitives who can tune in to your health and vital energy to identify sources of pain and areas that require attention and healing.

Longing = aching pain
Running, escaping = addiction
Rejecting = anorexia
Punishing = pain
Resisting, hardening = arteriosclerosis
Criticizing = arthritis
Smothering = asthma
Pinching = intestinal blockage

Retaining = bladder problems
Boiling = heart attack
Churning = stomach problems
Leaning = dependent

Go back and look at the words you and your partner chose to describe each other's energies that represent positive associations: expanding, glowing, soaring, giving, softening. These are the energies you will want to focus on and draw to you in your daily meditation practice. Focus on the chronic health problem you've targeted for attention and care. Now assign your positive energy to it. For example, let's take **churning = stomach problems.** Replace churning energy with caressing, opening, calming. When you catch yourself thinking churning thoughts—thoughts that turn over and over themselves in turmoil—replace them with caressing, opening, calming thoughts. It may help to build an affirmation around the energy you want to cultivate: *"Today, no matter what happens, I am calm, because I know that I am safe and secure."*

Chakras, the Tarot, and Life Energy

Your energy is your essence, the essential barometer of your health. In Eastern medicine, chakras are the energy centers in the body. They are believed to work as intake centers for the universal life force that surrounds us. Did you know that some people say they can see chakras? They describe them as whirling pools of light, each radiating its color. Each chakra spins at a different frequency. The root, or survival, chakra spins at the slowest frequency; the crown, or spirit, chakra spins at the fastest. When a chakra is closed, it stops taking in energy, and that imbalance is the beginning of disease.

Each of the seven chakras corresponds to an area of the body. All are connected through a channel of energy that ascends the center of the spine. One way to remember the chakras is to note that the colors of the chakras follow the same order as the colors of the rainbow, moving through the spectrum from red to violet.

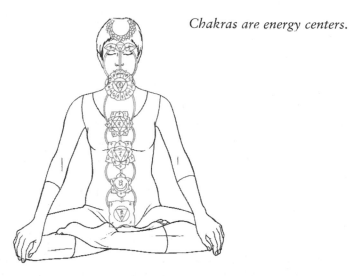

Chakras are energy centers.

Saturn ♄ chakra: The root. The root chakra is about survival—your basic needs. It governs your will to live and your physical vitality. It is located at the rectum and the base of the spine. When all is well with this chakra, you are grounded, secure, and confident, with the discipline and clarity of Saturn in your favor. When your root chakra is out of balance, you are deeply insecure, ruled by fear, and don't know where to turn when a crisis or challenge hits. Its color is red.

Jupiter ♃ chakra: Desire. This chakra governs your sexuality, your creativity, and your emotions. It also governs reproduction. It is located at the third and fourth vertebrae, just above the pubic bone. In balance, you can tap into the expansiveness of Jupiter for your creativity and imagination, and your sex life is satisfying. An out-of-balance second chakra may manifest itself in sexual obsession. Its color is orange.

Mars ♂ chakra: Power. This chakra rules your identity and your domain. A strong third chakra indicates good physical health. It is located in the solar plexus/navel area. The third chakra governs your ability to digest your emotions. When it's in balance, you will have the initiative and courage to achieve good deeds. Someone with a too-strong third chakra is greedy or power-hungry, while someone with a weak third chakra may be ruled by excessive emotions or be susceptible to illness. Its color is yellow.

Venus ♀ chakra: The heart. Yep, you guessed it. This one is about love—and kindness, compassion, forgiveness, and selflessness. When the heart chakra is open, you can attract true love. If it's out of balance, you will come across as cold-hearted—you are shutting it out. You will have trouble expressing love, and you will be jealous and selfish and you will think nobody loves you (how untrue!). Its color is green.

Mercury ☿ chakra: The throat. This is the chakra of expression—the words of truth, compassion, and wisdom. Located in the throat, this chakra is associated with the thyroid gland and lungs. When this chakra is strong, you can express your needs and get them met. When it's out of balance, you may be fearful of expressing your true feelings and keep silent—or you may be overly blunt and opinionated. Its color is blue.

Sun ☉ chakra: The third eye. This is the chakra of intuition— another way of seeing. It is located in the center of the forehead, a notch above the eyebrows and 1 inch beneath the skin. This is the chakra you activated with your partner in the previous Psychic Intuition exercise by using your ring finger, ruled by the Sun. The Sun chakra governs how you see the world and how you visualize yourself in it. At its ideal, this chakra helps develop visions for the good of all. When it's out of balance, your basic concept of the world is not based on reality, and your views are distorted. Its color is indigo.

Thousand-petal lotus chakra: The crown. This is the chakra of spirituality, bliss, and enlightenment. It is located at the crown, at the top of the skull. When this chakra is strong, you have a defined and vital spirituality. You have reached self-actualization. When it's weak, you are disconnected from spiritual experience. Its color is violet.

As you meditate on the chakras, one or more of them may resonate to your attention. You may have just emerged tattered and torn from a love relationship that ended bitterly, so you know already that your heart chakra is in need. Or you may have come through a round of a tough treatment regimen or a physically stressful period in your life, and feel your power and courage are diminished just when you require them the most. Tuning in to your chakras is simultaneously both subtle and obvious—there is the chakra that calls out loudly for attention, and the one that remains more elusive, the one you must pursue to release its energy. Use this Tarot Chakra Spread to gain insights into your chakra balance. To do this spread, lay out seven cards in a vertical column starting with card one at the base to signify the Saturn ♄ chakra and rising to card seven, signifying the lotus chakra. A client we will call Diane came to Arlene for a Tarot reading to ask *"What chakras are out of balance?"*

Diane's chakra reading.

Here's how Diane's cards relate to each chakra:

Chakra	Tarot Card	Keyword or Phrase
Saturn ♄ 1st—the root	2 of Swords R	Fragmented
Jupiter ♃ 2nd—desire	The World	Promise of fulfillment
Mars ♂ 3rd—power	Knight of Cups	New power
Venus ♀ 4th—heart	6 of Swords	Smoother waters ahead
Mercury ☿ 5th—throat	The Star	Expressing deeper wisdom
Sun ☉ 6th—third eye	Page of Pentacles	Study your intuition
Thousand- petal lotus 7th—crown	Queen of Cups R	Take a deep breath

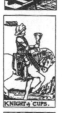

The two reversed cards immediately point to Diane's first and seventh chakras being out of balance, and that's where she should focus. The first chakra, remember, is about your basic survival needs, while the seventh is about spiritual needs. Diane should look to fostering the faith that grounds our energy in the very act of living, in survival.

The 2 of Swords reversed in her first chakra tells us Diane's basic self is fragmented. Note that the imagery is that of a blindfolded woman who has turned her back on the water. This card points to Diane's need for security and for getting in touch with her feelings. Because the Queen of Cups card, in the position of the seventh chakra, is about nurturing intuition, when it comes up reversed, it's a signal to take a deep breath, pause, reflect, and tap into your intuition. This card is telling Diane to get out of reactive mode in her spiritual life, harness her emotions, get quiet and go within, as she refills her cup of intuition.

The World card in Diane's second chakra points to attainment and self-actualization in the realm of sexuality and desire. This card promises fulfillment of all of Diane's desires if she can do the work presented by the other chakras.

The Knight of Cups in Diane's power chakra tells us issues of the heart are being brought to the fore for Diane in a powerful way. The Knight of Cups is a man of fortitude and genuine character who is offering an invitation. This could point to an opportunity coming Diane's way for her to respond differently than she has before, more centered and more in tune with her own power—as long as she works on the two chakras that are out of balance.

The 6 of Swords in the heart chakra shows that Diane is coming to the end of a difficult cycle in love. She is leaving the rough waters and heading toward calm seas. The Star in the expression chakra points to inspiration and hope—the expression of a new life through deeper wisdom.

The Page of Pentacles in the intuition chakra can indicate the need to study what is before you. The Page of Pentacles is an eager and bright student who acts upon what is learned. When this card comes up in the intuition chakra, it can tell you that the realm of intuition is not a mysterious world—it is safe to delve into it in a practical way.

How are *your* chakras balanced? Quietly, in a relaxed, seated meditation pose, breathe deeply and fully from your abdomen with seven deep breaths—one for each of the chakras. In each breath, send positive, releasing energy to resonate through the home of that chakra in your spine. Then take your Tarot deck, shuffle, and deal out the cards in the Chakra Spread. Meditate further on the images and potential meanings of each and record your insights in your Intuitive Arts notebook.

War and Peace: Mars ♂ in Your Birth Chart

The most toxic emotion may be anger, but psychologists say that anger isn't the real emotion. Anger is often a mask for deep hurt, and it is the emotion that we may delay dealing with the most. But unresolved anger can come back and haunt us in ways that are life-threatening. All of us deal with anger differently. To see how you deal with anger, look at where Mars ♂ appears in your astrological birth chart. If your chart shows you have a tendency to a fiery temper, that's not all she wrote. The placement of Mars in your chart doesn't indicate destiny, but rather gives clues on how to handle your anger, to learn new behaviors. Here's a look, sign by sign, at Mars's influence on your temper.

Mars ♂ in Aries ♈. You can be aggressive and headstrong, but you can also be courageous and tell the truth. You don't let anything stand in your way, so you can accomplish a lot. Sometimes, however, you need to let go—not to knock down the obstacles in your path, but to use finesse to go around them. You can be attached to your way of doing things. Your challenge will be to try to understand others' points of view, when you are so certain your own is the right and only way. Ask yourself "Do I want to be right, or do I want to be happy?" Or ask yourself "What can this (fill in the blank: person, situation, place, thing) teach me?"

Mars ♂ in Taurus ♉. You are persistent in an earthy, unfolding, and quiet way—the opposite of the Aries ♈ push. Your stolid patience can seem like stalling to others around you, but we see it as a true-blue commitment to reach your goals. You can seem immovable and draw the ire of the Mutable signs around you. Your challenge will be to let yourself make little changes, to take one step closer to your partner's point of view. It may be hard for others to pick up when you are angry, because you are so methodical and will direct your expression of anger toward the dogged pursuit of your desires.

Mars ♂ in Gemini ♊. You are quicksilver, always considering, acting, expressing, and changing course to satisfy your needs. You decide easily, are precise with language, and nurture resourcefulness, which can serve you well in conflicts. You get to the heart of the matter quickly, even if it hurts. Because you're quick to move on, the injury is not deep and lasting, and it doesn't fester. Your challenge is that you will seem restless to your partner and your friends. They will find you mercurial, often unpredictable, and if they have a different style of expressing anger, they may have difficulty trusting you.

Mars ♂ in Cancer ♋. You internalize, protecting your feelings, which sometimes can manifest as passive-aggressive behavior. But because you are so intuitive and sensitive, you may be so tuned in with the person you are in conflict with that you work out solutions in your indirect way that are to the best benefit of both of you. You have taken into account your friend's feelings in a deep and knowing way—without a lot of overt communication. Your protective energy around your feelings means they are hard to express, and you can get defensive when probed, and that could lead to angry exchanges with loved ones. Your challenge is developing an open, two-way dialogue when working through conflicts.

Mars ♂ in Leo ♌. Fire! Fire! Fire! Mars fire flares in Leo. Your passion can get you into trouble, because you can be passionate about

125

everything—and many of those things don't matter quite *so* much. Your challenge will be knowing when to let go, and letting go can feel like such a huge compromise that you feel like you are not being true to yourself. You must still let go. When you are in conflict with more subtle Mars types, you may completely miss their anger because they are not as direct in expressing it as you are! "You cared about that?" you may wonder in complete surprise.

Mars ♂ in Virgo ♍. You are levelheaded and meticulous. You tend to analyze your emotions before you give yourself a chance to feel them. Your challenge is that you are so good at separating yourself from your emotions, you might bury your anger. You might have a tendency to stew. If you have a life partner, he or she probably has quickly sensed this and gets tuned in to when you stew. You value being clever and shrewd, keeping your head, so much that your partner and your friends will need to encourage you to be blunt sometimes. While your perfectionist nature may express itself in patience that goes beyond the call of duty, you may find yourself lacking patience in dealing with the perceived flaws of others.

Mars ♂ in Libra ♎. You know right from wrong, and are balanced and fair-minded (or strive to be), with a high desire for beauty and harmony. Your desire for harmony means you get angry very infrequently. But your sense of justice can sometimes lead to outrage. And righteous outrage is what it is when you are angry. You want your relationships to be equal and fair. When they're not—and nobody said life was fair— you may have a tendency to pout or brood rather than work it all out. After all, you want harmony. Your challenge is you may want it so much that you hold back expressing your concerns when a relationship is out of balance.

Mars ♂ in Scorpio ♏. You are intense and like fulfilling your desire. Mars in Scorpio can be enterprising or intractable, mesmerizing or obsessive—or all of the above. Mars in Scorpio is powerful and charismatic, and your anger, when it's expressed, is potent. When used wisely, it can be a transforming anger, the kind that brings up a conflict and lifts a relationship to a whole new level. But the transforming anger can leave casualties in its wake, and so you must be conscious of holding back the sting of your words, lest you say something you will regret just as powerfully later.

Mars ♂ in Sagittarius ♐. You are the daring and far-sighted adventurer. You can be open and honest—a little *too* honest at times. You may not be sensitive to the piercing arrows of your words when you are angry. Always, your anger is about taking a relationship to an intrepid, new level. It comes from a desire to improve on and discover the possibilities of a relationship, but others don't always see it that way. You rarely hold back your anger, so your challenge is to be more sensitive about snapping that bow. Think about how your target must feel when the arrow hits.

Mars ♂ in Capricorn ♑. You have a plan. Your anger, when expressed, is responsible and patient, controlled. You are willing to work hard on working through your anger. Your anger is never lightning fast, nor is it a storm that passes quickly. When you are angry about something, you want to work through it, and you will follow solutions through all the way to the end. Your challenge is that you are *so* wedded to your goal-oriented process. You will be thrown off balance by those with Mars in signs that let all their anger come out in unpredictable (at least to you!) ways. You don't need to take it all so seriously. Some of us are just blowing off steam.

Mars ♂ in Aquarius ♒. Your knack for remaining aloof from the crowd means you rarely get angry. Most things just don't bother you, because in the cosmic scheme of things, getting angry about them is trivial. When you are angry, it may arise from impatience with those who don't resonate to your intellectual, airy approach. You just don't get it about getting down in the muck and working it out. Your anger is high-minded. Yet, when you hit a conflict, your approach is progressive and inventive. You look to the future and don't hold on to the past. Those in close relationships with you will find, for the most part, that yours is a healthy anger, because you always want to turn it into a positive.

Mars ♂ in Pisces ♓. You tend to go with the flow, which can mean that you are often not in touch with your anger. You may be so self-sacrificing that you don't realize when you are giving too much. You often take on other people's emotional burdens, and don't even know to get angry about it. Your tendency to escape can mask your anger. Thus, when you are angry, you might not know where it came from. You may deal with it in an unfocused way—or at least it may appear that way to the subject of your anger! To use your anger well, Mars in Pisces can channel it into compassion and move toward higher consciousness.

As you can see, some of the signs show a tendency to hold in anger in ways that can be destructive to you over time. Others show that the way you unleash anger can destroy others—pushing love away from you. All of the Mars ♂ placements in the astrological signs present a choice. You can fall into the worst tendencies of your Mars sign or you can use your challenges to deal with your anger in healthful ways.

Retrogrades ℞: Re-Doing, Releasing, and Healing

If you suffer from chronic health problems, you may find progress is slow. You may post victories, only to see them slip away and find yourself right back where you started. This can really get you down. If you understand the role of retrograde ℞ planets in your astrological birth chart, however, you can work with the energies of the universe. A retrograde planet is one that appears to be moving backward. When the universe is guiding you forward in direct motion, you can gain the most ground in health through action. When the energy of the universe is spinning the other way, you will tap into the energy of introspection, self-renewal, and healing.

There are two ways of talking about retrogrades—a personal retrograde and a transiting retrograde. A personal retrograde in your birth chart means that planet looked as if it were moving backward in its orbit around the Sun at the time of your birth. A personal retrograde affects only you and gives insight into what you came into this world equipped to re-do. A transiting retrograde affects us all. It reflects what is happening in the moment and calls upon us all to re-do or rethink the energy of the planet that is in transiting retrograde.

First, we take a look at your personal retrogrades—the planets that were retrograde in your astrological chart at the time of your birth. They give you insight into the kind of healing work you need to do and how that planet will influence your choices and your actions around health. Some of your retrograde planets may comfort you in the knowledge that this is your style of working with your health; others retrograde planets may present more of a challenge. Note that some of the "assignments" of personal retrogrades are pretty tall orders—look at Pluto ♀. In the case of Neptune ♆ retrograde ℞, failing to heed the call can have damaging consequences for your physical health. The Saturn ♄ retrograde ℞ challenge is in learning to say no, while the Mars ♂ retrograde ℞ challenge is not to punish yourself with your own anger.

If This Planet Is Retrograde ℞ in Your Birth Chart ...	It Means
Mercury ☿	You are an iconoclast—you think differently from the rest of us. You are quite capable of new perspectives on your health, and on a global scale, on how our society defines

**If This Planet Is
Retrograde ℞ in
Your Birth Chart ...**   **It Means**

wellness, treats people who are disabled or frail, and approaches health remedies.

Because Mercury is the planet of communication, when its energy is turned the other direction, it means you might take a little longer to process news about your health.

Venus ♀

You tend to go against the grain of aesthetics and social values, finding beauty in things very different from those usually considered beautiful. In relationships, it may be more difficult to show your love outwardly. A health crisis can make you reconsider relationships around you. Working on expressing your love may prove to be a healing source for you.

Mars ♂

Your hard-charging warrior energy is turned inward. Your anger may be turned inward as well, and it may affect your health. Work on finding healthy ways to release your anger.

Jupiter ♃

You may have unconventional philosophies, faith, and cultural values. Once you become comfortable with your singular path, you will have a strong and intense faith that can guide you through rocky times with your health. Know that you must seek inner growth first to see your unique path, before you can direct your growth toward the community. If not, your health may suffer because you deplete your energy and lose your center.

Saturn ♄

You may not know how to say "no," and have problems setting limits. You may take on too much and deplete yourself. If you don't resolve health problems by giving them enough attention or working on prevention, Saturn may bring a recurrence. A Saturn retrograde may also indicate genetic health problems.

If This Planet Is Retrograde ℞ in Your Birth Chart ...	It Means
Uranus ♅	Uranus's natural desire to reform is even more pronounced in a retrograde Uranus. Your subconscious strongly influences your motivations; as a result, your physical health can be affected by any early childhood trauma or repressed emotion.
Neptune ♆	You are called to a spiritual journey that tests your faith. A test of faith can trigger a health crisis—or vice versa. A health crisis can set you on a quest toward enlightenment that you have been delaying. Delay at your potential peril—spiritually bereft retrograde Neptune may seek solace in substance abuse to achieve a false sense of spiritual bliss.
Pluto ♀	You seek to transform—yourself, your health, your environment, the world at large. A health crisis can move you to reexamine yourself. It's your life mission to be reborn to new ways of approaching health. You have always been blessed with the unique ability to see how your behaviors affect the health of the world, and your relationships with people near and far.

We look at transiting retrogrades ℞ when we are looking at the patterns of our everyday effort to be healthy in body, mind, and spirit. Knowing where the energy of the universe is directed can guide you in knowing whether to advance or retreat. A good source for mapping out retrogrades for the year ahead is an astrological ephemeris. Another: the *Celestial Calendars* by Jim Maynard—and they are pocket-size and portable. Here's a quick trip through the transiting retrogrades.

Transiting Retrograde ℞	When	It's a Time of ...
Mercury ☿	*3 times a year, about 3 weeks each time*	Communication and transportation delays and mix-ups; excellent time to study and learn about new healing methods

Transiting Retrograde ℞	When	It's a Time of ...
Venus ♀	*6 weeks out of a 584-day cycle*	Looking and listening deeply to reevaluate personal relationships, including your relationship with yourself
Mars ♂	*9 to 10 weeks out of a 26-month cycle*	Learning to cope with anger, heal old wounds, and foster beneficial action
Jupiter ♃	*4 months every 13 months*	Applying boisterous optimism to internal contemplation before returning to share insights with the world
Saturn ♄	*4½ months every 12½ months*	Reconsidering any kind of structure and exploring how you use power and relate to authority
Uranus ♅	*5 months every year*	Exploring how you are preventing or encouraging change—realign your personal goals and your community service goals
Neptune ♆	*5 to 6 months every year*	Looking at your Jungian shadow side, the dark and emotional places you fear within yourself; a time to meditate and receive intuitive answers about your health
Pluto ♇	*5 months every year*	Reevaluate your spiritual growth and transformation to go to a deeper level of healing

The Jupiter Track: The Role of Optimism

Optimists live longer. In a recent study conducted at the Mayo Clinic in Rochester, Minnesota, researchers tracked 529 women and 310 men for 3 decades, using the MMPI (Minnesota Multiphasic Personality Inventory) to sort out who was an optimist and who was a pessimist. You'll be interested to know that 124 subjects were classified as optimistic and 197 as pessimistic, but most of them—518—exhibited a mix. We are complex beings. Of the 839 subjects, 200 died during the course of the study. When researchers compared subjects' expected life spans with their actual life spans, they found that pessimists were 19 percent more likely to die early. On the other hand, optimists lived significantly longer than expected.

A study that tracked Harvard University graduates found the pessimists among them were more likely to suffer from poor health at ages 45 through 60. Another study found that optimists are more likely to seek medical care—and get well. Still another study of 238 patients battling cancer revealed that younger pessimistic subjects (aged 30 to 59 years) were at an increased risk of death, compared with their optimistic peers.

Even better, one study found not only that optimism protects your health and longevity, it can reverse health problems. Barbara Frederickson, winner of the Templeton Positive Psychology Prize, found in laboratory-based studies that positive emotions such as joy, contentment, and love can *undo* the detrimental effects of negative emotions on the cardiovascular system.

Let's see how the cockeyed optimist of the cosmos is influencing your health. Meet the planet Jupiter ♃. Jupiter in your astrological birth chart is expansive, generous, and vital. Jupiter is about opportunity; Jupiter helps you see the possibilities in life. Jupiter calls upon you to use your higher mind. With Jupiter, we all have the potential to tap into the healing power of positive thinking—just in different ways.

Jupiter ♃ In	Its Influence	How to Tap Into It
Aries ♈	A childlike curiosity, courage	Engage in child play, creative arts, new ventures.
Taurus ♉	Abundance, wealth (both material and spiritual), steady growth	Look back and see your progress in increments; reflect on past and present abundance; look ahead and map out a steady course; periodically reflect on how far you have come.
Gemini ♊	Good luck, finding yourself in fortunate circumstances	Recognize your savvy and quick-thinking skill; see the serendipity in your life. Travel.
Cancer ♋	Good natured, good sense of humor, positive outlook	Laugh. Gather others around you who make you laugh. Listen to others who have similar stories. Family connections can point you to nurturing your inner child.

Jupiter ♃ In	Its Influence	How to Tap Into It
Leo ♌	Sees life on a grand scale and encourages others to do the same; kind, lionhearted	Through giving, gathering many people around you. A Leo in Jupiter is the kind of person who can make a hospital visit a party.
Virgo ♍	Growth felt as a sacred duty, and applies precision to the process	When you can see your course mapped out in small, pragmatic steps, you will have the confidence to step forward.
Libra ♎	Facilitates, looks to establish partnerships	Form alliances with others around your health; surround yourself with positive people. A Libra in Jupiter will have aromatherapy candles everywhere.
Scorpio ♏	Faith applied with powerful intent	A challenge. Nothing gets you fired up more than someone who says you don't have it in you.
Sagittarius ♐	Carpe diem!	Look ahead and visualize the healthy you in the future. When an opportunity comes in the form of good advice from a friend or a health practitioner who is ready to tackle this with you, seize it!
Capricorn ♑	Goal setting with strong ethics	You need to feel that you are are going about your health problems in an honorable way. You will stay loyal to your providers and supporters, and you need their loyalty, too.
Aquarius ♒	Advocacy for humanity's best destiny, evolution through innovation	Devote your energy to a cause that helps others. Create an "extended" family, a Community family of the heart.
Pisces ♓	Emotional tides, high and low; compassionate truth	Engage in creative activities that stimulate your imagination and plumb your emotional depths; analyze your dream life.

The Hope Card: Tarot's Star

For our final destination, we arrive at Tarot's Star, a personal favorite of Carolyn's. The Star card is the first card in the last segment of the journey of the Major Arcana. The last five cards of the Major Arcana represent the rewards of the life lessons at the end of the Fool's journey. Let's take this card out of your Tarot deck and use it for a meditation.

In the Star card, a pure luminescent woman pours one urn of water onto the land, our physical world, while releasing the other into the watery realm of emotions into which she also dips her own foot. Above her is an eight-pointed star that symbolizes the glow of inspiration and spiritual enlightenment. The seven smaller stars represent wisdom the woman has used in her life journey to this place. The Star nurtures serene hope, faith, and the desire to manifest the joy and bliss we know lies beneath the surface of all that is seen and unseen.

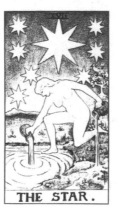

Tarot's Star lights the way to well-being.

Take a few moments to meditate on the promise of this card. What is it telling you about your health? What is your vision for your health? Bring the picture of the most healthful you into focus. Wrap yourself lovingly in the courage and hope of this card. See yourself giving and receiving love. Spend a few moments describing you at your best in your Intuitive Arts notebook.

Looking for Bliss in Your Birth Chart

You can look within your birth chart to find the natural origins of all of your potential bliss. Unlocking the secret of your own natural path to bliss is the beginning of the road back to vitality. To show you how to do that, we'll take a look at the birth chart of the Dalai Lama. Note that he is a Cancer Sun ♋ ☉, meaning that compassion and empathy define his core self. With a Virgo Moon ♍ ☽, he is intuitively attuned to the sacred patterns of the universe and the quest for spiritual perfection. But look closer, and you'll find Mars ♂ in Libra ♎. The influence of fair-minded and balanced Libra is the perfect antidote to the warring nature of Mars, and this reveals a lot about the Dalai Lama's timeless teachings on the ways of peace. His Mars in Libra can bring out the "negotiator of peace and diplomacy" in the face of disaster or threats.

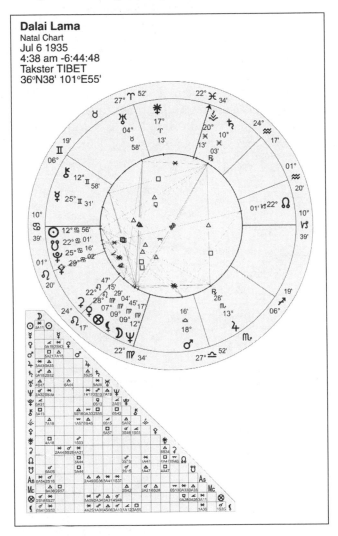

The Dalai Lama's birth chart.

135

Also note that Jupiter ♃ is in Scorpio ♏, which we described earlier as "faith with powerful intent." If that doesn't describe the Dalai Lama, then Tibet is a flat, featureless desert! The pairing of Jupiter in Scorpio is potent, an unleashing of the transformative power that comes when we truly believe and can let go. But also note that Jupiter is in retrograde ℞, which means that the Dalai Lama's unwavering commitment to his beliefs and path of personal growth would gather strength later in life as others came to see the infinite wisdom of his choices. His Jupiter retrograde would indicate an unconscious desire and drive to complete not only his personal growth but to help others attain the same bliss and contentment.

You, too, are equipped, in ways you might have never known, to find the joy despite the struggles with your health. Take a few moments now to locate the indicators in your chart—Mars ♂, Jupiter ♃, and the retrogrades ℞. Make some notes about times in your life when your natural skills have carried you through conflicts and challenges. How might you tap into those skills again?

chapter 7

When There Isn't a Clear Fix

The Hanged Man and the Devil release your demons
Falling from Tarot's Tower
You say you want a revolution: Uranus ♅
A new place: Your Saturn ♄ return
Phases of grieving: Use Astrology to chart them
From Death to the Magician
Pluto ♀ power

Sometimes the magic answer for your health problems remains elusive. Or the answer isn't what you want to hear. The answer may be that you have a health problem you will have to live with for the rest of your life. What do you do when there is no clear fix? How can you redirect your efforts toward healing and acceptance, embracing the beauty of your life? Many who have faced the paradox of a health problem that won't go away have found the courage to embrace it as a gift. It takes them to uncharted places. In this chapter, we use Tarot to help you discover how to unleash the transformative healing represented in the Hanged Man, the Devil, and the Tower cards. We turn to rebellious Uranus for liberation and inspiration. We use the suit of Wands, the Death card, and plenty of Pluto power to help you tap into your personal strength. As Mother Superior tells young Maria in The Sound of Music, "Sometimes you have to look for your life." We use the Intuitive Arts to help you find that life is always beautiful.

The Hanged Man and the Devil: Release Your Demons

A health crisis can push you to take a good, hard, honest look at your health. It may be the *only* catalyst that forces you to do so. We all know someone who has unhealthy habits and knows better but keeps eating poorly (and/or overeating) or smoking or not exercising until the blinding flash of a life crisis forces change. People with chronic health problems such as back pain, or depression, or Epstein-Barr virus often "soldier on," coping resignedly for years without relief—until the day comes when they can't live with the situation anymore, when they say, "This must change." It may take a loss or threat of loss to get you working earnestly on healing. Maybe your life partner or a family member intervenes, or maybe you are hanging by a thread at work.

Enter Tarot's Hanged Man. This Major Arcana card represents the turning point. The Hanged Man is not who you would think at first glance—a criminal shamed and prosecuted, receiving punishment for a crime. This hanged man is not dead (remember the guy in *Monty Python's Holy Grail*, "I'm *not* dead"), with a noose around his neck. This hanged man is suspended by one foot. You could say he is hanging by a thread.

This card represents the point of releasing all those things that are holding you back. Notice that the Hanged Man is not in distress. Instead, his facial expression is one of calm and around his head glows a *nimbus,* a medieval symbol of blessed protection. This Hanged Man is prepared to make sacrifices for the higher good. The Hanged Man surrenders his ego and submits to a higher wisdom. By accepting his situation, he opens himself up to a new realm of possibilities. When this card comes up in a reading, it's a signal that while you have not left your current situation, you are ready to evolve spiritually and move in a new direction.

Meditate on the Hanged Man. Ask yourself some hard questions: Is there anything in your life that you are clinging to—people, beliefs, routines, places? Is there a sacrifice—or just simply a *big* change—you know you need to make? Why don't you want to let go? What are you afraid of? Do you feel you are hanging by a thread? What do you imagine would happen if the thread were to dissolve? Would you change careers? Move to a different place? Distance yourself from loved ones? If you let go, would you lose control? Would feelings come out that you have been trying to suppress or deny? What are you risking if you express them? Will you lose your dignity? Will you have to rely on others? On yourself? Imagine what may seem the "worst-case" scenario and what you would do if it were to happen. Now imagine letting go of some of the things that are hurting you. Imagine all of those fears dissolving. Imagine the sigh of relief when you no longer have to tie yourself to this reality.

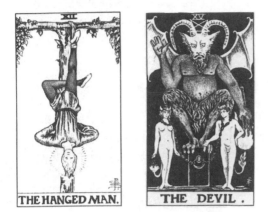

The Hanged Man represents releasing the old, painful reality and submitting to a higher wisdom. The Devil represents making friends with your life's dark shadows.

If you struggle with a chronic health problem, a permanent disability, or a life-diminishing or life-threatening disease or condition, you may feel as if you are in bondage. If you struggle with lifestyle habits that undermine your efforts at health, you may feel you are fighting something bigger than yourself. Certainly Carolyn understands this. Her father struggled with his weight all of his life. When he died unexpectedly at 62, he was obese and had massive heart disease that had gone undetected on EKG tests. Her father was a Virgo Sun sign ♍ ☉ with a Pisces Moon ♓ ☽, and Pisces is a sign susceptible to the lure of addiction. For Carolyn's father, as for too many people these days, the addiction was food. In his last days at the hospital, as he struggled to catch a breath and hold on to his courage and good-natured sense of humor (picture Carolyn's father as Jupiter incarnate), he said, "I've had about as much of this as I can take."

You may also feel you are struggling with demons that plague your best efforts at health. The constant effort to wrestle with these relentless demons can tire you, and make them seem bigger and more formidable. In the throes of the struggle, you may not even be aware of what they are. These demons appear like stealthy intruders in the night—monstrous shadows in a dark room. You may lose sight of the people around you who are poised to clobber your demons with a 2×4. It may feel like there is nowhere to turn.

Asking the Tarot some courageous questions using the Devil card can help dispel those demons. Like turning on the light in a dark room, the shadows are illuminated. The Devil card can point to what holds us in chains. It can show us our temptations and our obsessions. You have heard the expression, "The Devil made me do it." Indeed, it may seem like someone else is in control, tempting you to indulge in the very behaviors that traumatize your efforts at health.

Go ahead, ask Tarot's Devil: What are my weaknesses? Why do I succumb to these temptations? What are my obsessions? Why do I turn to them? *When* do I turn to them? What is out of control in my life? What seems bigger than my efforts to rein it in? What does it seem like I can't help but do?

Let's do a Seven-Card Spread using the Hanged Man and the Devil card as the focal points. Start by choosing one card from the Tarot deck you feel best represents your feelings about your health situation right now. Place the Hanged Man to the left of this card and the Devil to the right. Shuffle the deck and place two cards to the left of the Hanged Man; card one shows what you need to release, while card two reveals what your demons are. Place two cards to the right of the Devil; card six shows what must be done to let go, while card 7 reveals your first step in shedding your demons.

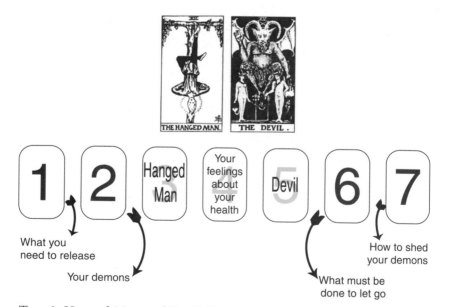

Tarot's Hanged Man and Devil show you where your demons are and help you to release them.

Revolution: The Tower and Uranus ♅

If your health challenges have pushed you to the point of saying, "I can't do this anymore," it may be time for a revolution. You may be in so much pain or just so tired of battling your health problems that you are past the point of caring what catches in fire on your life and falls burning to the ground.

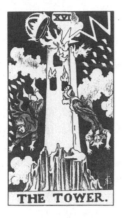

The Tower card represents the bolt from the blue.

In the Tower card, a lightning bolt sets the spire aflame, literally blowing the lid off in the symbol of the king's crown. Two people jump from the tower to certain death (or so it seems) on the jagged rocks. Flames lick the windows, smoke billows, and raindrops fall in the shape of *yod,* the Hebrew letter that symbolizes the hand of God. If you picked the Tower card in Chapter 1 when we associated cards to biblical images, and we listed the Tower of Babel, you were right on. This is the card of change, much like the African goddess Oya, who brings both destruction and potential with her sudden storms.

The Tower signals feelings or events that signify a point of no return. You may feel like the people in the tower when you receive an unexpected diagnosis. Or if you have been dealing with a diagnosis, it can signal release from your situation. The Tower can point to a dramatic shift in perception about your illness. You can even use the Tower card to *direct* your thoughts to inviting the unexpected, cathartic change into your life. No matter what your situation, meditating on Tarot's Tower can help you understand that shaking up your reality is not always the *worst* thing that can happen. The moment may seem cataclysmic, but there is also the moment that follows and the potential for creating a new, more successful, sustainable, and enduring way of being. That's how Tarot's Tower leads us to Astrology's planet, Uranus ♅.

Uranus ♅ in your astrological chart is the liberator. Uranus represents a breakthrough—and breakthrough is what we want here, isn't it? Uranus is about inviting bold new ways of thinking, the energy of change, growth, freedom, and expansion. Uranus releases you from the "status quo." Uranus challenges outdated beliefs, causing you to transcend your reality in search of innovative, wholly new ways of thinking and being. With Uranus, the solution you find may be one you have not yet considered, or it may represent a medical technology breakthrough that is today unimagined. It takes Uranus 84 years to complete its orbit around the Sun and 7 years to move from one astrological sign to another. Inventive Aquarius ♒ is its natural sign, and that is where Uranus ♅ could be found from 1996 to 2003. Uranus moved into intuitive Pisces ♓ in 2003 and will stay there until 2011.

Uranus ♅ is in Aries ♈ for people born 1927 to 1934/35. Combine liberation with a pioneering spirit, and you have Uranus in Aries. You find it easy and natural to abandon the status quo and explore uncharted territory. You may be the first to volunteer for a clinical trial in a new treatment or opt for a homeopathic regimen.

Uranus ♅ is in Taurus ♉ for people born 1934/35 to 1941/42. Your willpower will get you through the unleashing of sudden and unexpected changes. You can be steady as a rock while the world is catching on fire around you. Knowing that you have a strong inner fortitude can equip you as you navigate a changing landscape, upon receiving a diagnosis or asking the universe for a whole new way of looking at your illness. Your greatest challenge may be in letting go of material things as you invite new ways of approaching your health.

Uranus ♅ is in Gemini ♊ for people born 1941/42 to 1948/49. Your approach to liberating change is all intellectual. You have a powerful ability to direct your thoughts to change. For you, it can be mind over matter. You can envision a creative approach, and you can move quickly. You can thrive on keeping a journal about your illness and directing your thoughts on the life you visualize post-treatment. Barbara Kline Hammond, author of the book *Cancer's Gifts,* is a Uranus in Gemini who turned her healing efforts into communication. Her company has a decidedly Uranus name: Breakthru Communications.

Uranus ♅ is in Cancer ♋ for people born 1948/49 to 1955/56. You are well equipped for emotional revolution, and open to nontraditional ideas about home and family. You seek emotional freedom, and you chart new waters in your approach to your relationships with friends and family. You may from a young age have called your parents by

their first names rather than Mom or Dad, because you rejected the idea
that parents are authority figures and at an early age you saw them as
people. You may be good friends with your own adult children. If you
have Uranus in Cancer, you can draw upon these qualities during
a time of a transforming illness. Your innovative approach to family
and community may lead you to start a residential treatment facility or
nontraditional healing communities, creating new family and support
systems for those facing illness.

Uranus ♅ is in Leo ♌ for people born 1955/56 to 1961/62. Combine
fierce determination and creativity with desire for liberation, and you
have Uranus in Leo. With Uranus in Leo, you are more than willing to
cast aside ideas that aren't working for your best health. Your instincts
quickly tell you what will work best, and you can trust them as you
embrace new approaches. You may turn to creative expression—art,
poetry, pottery, beading, visual journaling—in releasing the complex
emotions around the changes your illness has brought in your life.

Uranus ♅ is in Virgo ♍ for people born 1961/62 to 1968/69. Tap
into the reforming qualities of Virgo and combine with the breakthrough energy of Uranus, and you can have real lasting change. Your
analytical, discriminating approach can keep the wildness of Uranus in
check. You are naturally oriented to the sacred healing connection of
humanity and the Earth, so it is easy for you to embrace organic foods
and natural remedies.

Uranus ♅ is in Libra ♎ for people born 1968/69 to 1974/75. Your
desire for radical changes won't just be limited to your personal health.
You will want to effect social change for the benefit of all who are challenged by your illness. You are likely to be the first to start a support
group or become a fund-raiser for a cause. Your strength in forming
partnerships means it will get off the ground quickly. You may help
your own health by starting a new organization that supports research.
You are all about big-picture solutions. Your Libra penchant for
beauty may lead you to developing or promoting products that enhance
well-being—aromatherapy, natural cosmetics, or flower essences.

Uranus ♅ is in Scorpio ♏ for people born 1974/75 to 1981. The
power of this pairing is cosmic! Scorpio, the sign of regeneration, is
paired with the revolutionary powers of Uranus. Your illness may have
you just now discovering your innate powerful capacity for change. The
potency of the Scorpion can have far-reaching effects. Your challenge
will be in letting go. Whatever you must release will feel like a death,
like an unforgettable fire. But from the sparks buried in the ashes, you
will be unleashing a healing fire, a new heat, a personal alchemy.

Uranus ♅ is in Sagittarius ♐ for people born 1981 to 1988. Your optimistic, adventurous nature will lift you through change. Your illness may guide you in seeking reforms in the realms of organized religion, the legal system, and education. It may guide you in leading others in new spiritual practices, or in changing laws in your state to allow medical freedom of choice. You may speak out against the cultural messages we receive and believe about illness—after all, we are a culture that fears frailty. Wherever you direct your focus, you will speak your convictions strongly and truthfully.

Uranus ♅ is in Capricorn ♑ for people born 1905 to 1912 and 1988 to 1995/96. You focus your efforts on planning how to replace old, obsolete, or unworkable constructions and structures with new ones. You are the person who will take on the HMO approach to health care or the insurance companies that keep your health treatments tied up in red tape. You have a powerful ability to concentrate your energy on building better situations.

Uranus ♅ is in Aquarius ♒ for people born 1912 to 1919/20 and 1995/96 to 2003. This natural pairing (Uranus rules Aquarius) is characterized by innovation, let's say, *universal* change. You are equipped with an unwavering desire to transform reality in a positive, progressive way. You are democratic in process, so you will be concerned with listening to all voices and developing a consensus.

Uranus ♅ is in Pisces ♓ for people born 1919/20 to 1927 and 2003 to 2010/11. Those born under this pairing will approach personal and physical change through intuition. Theirs won't necessarily be a cognitive approach: They may tap into their dream world for visions of change, and will have strong and natural psychic awareness. Because of the Pisces challenge with addiction, this pairing may bring radical approaches in wrestling with our demons. Because of the Pisces association with Jesus and sacrifice, this combination means you will be adept at sacrifice and release. A whole new generation of Uranus in Pisces is about to be born in the next seven years. Imagine what the future holds!

For more clues about the arena in which your Uranus energy can bring about breakthroughs, look at your astrological chart to see in which house Uranus appears. The astrological house in which Uranus appears is certain to guarantee an unconventional approach to that issue, and it points to a crisis occurring in that area of your life at some point in your lifetime. The purpose for the crisis: To lift your soul consciousness to a whole new level of awareness. Uranus brings about the turning point in life.

Before a horse-riding accident that left him paralyzed (May 27, 1995), Christopher Reeve played the embodiment of strength, vitality, and invincibility: Superman. Since then, he has radically changed our ideas about frailty, serving as a spokesperson for paraplegics and vowing that he will walk again. He and his wife have talked openly about how his disability has strained their marriage, but it has lifted them to a new level of love for each other. A look at his birth chart shows that Reeve is a Libra Sun ♎ ☉ sign with a Sagittarius Moon ♐ ☽ and Leo ♌ ascendant.

Chris's Uranus ♅ falls in Cancer ♋, which enlightens us about his sensitive and innovative approach to his disability. With a harmonious Libra Sun and liberating Uranus in Cancer, it's easy to see why he is uniquely poised to be the voice of compassion and inspiration for paraplegics. With a proud Leo ♌ rising, it must have been very hard for Chris to have his body fail him and not be the picture of perfect health. But it also indicates that his constitution and determination are very strong and that he is oriented to be a leader who will educate the public. Uranus's home house is the 11th house, the house of hopes and dreams, and that's where Reeve's Uranus appears. This indicates he has a strong interest in humanitarian concerns—and he will be able to change his life goals unexpectedly, finding a new path as he needs to.

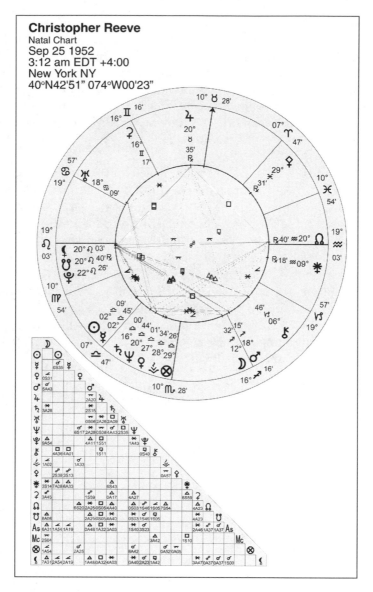

Christopher Reeve
Natal Chart
Sep 25 1952
3:12 am EDT +4:00
New York NY
40°N42'51" 074°W00'23"

Christopher Reeve's birth chart.

A New Path: Your Saturn ♄ Return

About 28 to 30 years after you are born, Saturn returns to the same point in your chart that it was at your birth. This happens again around age 58 to 60 and, if you are lucky enough to live that long, at 90. It's called a Saturn ♄ return, and when Saturn comes back, it's time for a life progress report. You will assess what is working and what isn't. How you come out of this struggle determines how you will plan for your future. During a Saturn return, people often experience life shifts. They may change careers—or spouses—or they may relocate. If you are experiencing health problems during a Saturn return, it may be that your illness is directing you to close one chapter of your life and begin another. To get a chart showing your Saturn return, you will need to consult an astrologer such as Arlene.

Here are some of the characteristics of a Saturn return:

☙ Certain dreams or goals lose importance in your life.

☙ You may commit to an exciting new challenge, one that will unfold over the years to come and influence your future choices.

☙ You will go about building a new, firm foundation for your life.

☙ Once that's in place, you will start having fun again. With a new foundation in place, you can feel carefree.

A Saturn return isn't always an earth-shaking life change. It's about evaluating your life to that point. If you have done your work up until the time of its return, you will be rewarded. In this chart, the outer wheel shows Christopher Reeve's Saturn return, while the inner wheel is Reeve's birth chart. Note that in both, Saturn has returned to Libra ♎, within a few degrees of the point it was at Reeve's birth. At the time of Reeve's Saturn return, he found himself at the height of his popularity in the *Superman* films, the first of which was released in late 1978. Those films—four in a series culminating in 1987—forever etched him in memory as the "Man of Steel": strong, charismatic, and heroic. For Reeve, his Saturn return is the culmination of devoting himself to his love of acting. Note that his 6th house of work and health has Capricorn ♑ on the cusp. Because Saturn is the ruler of Capricorn, this indicates the focus of his Saturn return would be on work and health. For Reeve, discipline paid off!

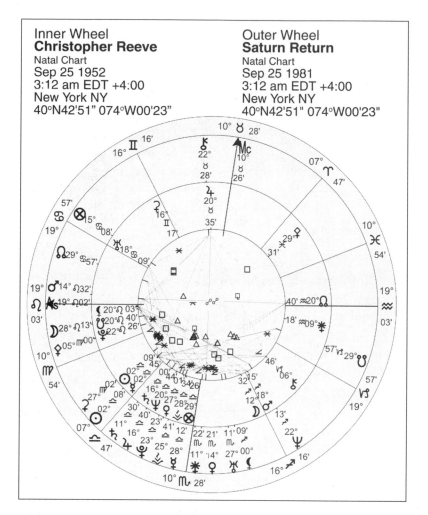

Inner Wheel
Christopher Reeve
Natal Chart
Sep 25 1952
3:12 am EDT +4:00
New York NY
40°N42'51" 074°W00'23"

Outer Wheel
Saturn Return
Natal Chart
Sep 25 1981
3:12 am EDT +4:00
New York NY
40°N42'51" 074°W00'23"

Christopher Reeve's Saturn ♄ return.

Finding Acceptance in Grief Through the Intuitive Arts

Living with an illness can bring up all sorts of questions. You may be able to look back and see clearly the habits and indulgences that led to your body's breakdown. Self-blame is painful (and not always helpful), so you may turn away and look for someone or something else to blame. When you condemn that "guilty" entity directly or just direct your inner energy negatively in that direction, you deny yourself the potential positive healing aspects that the relationship might offer if you are willing to look for them—however impossible that possibility may seem to you now. When that happens, you feel isolated, and you may even direct your anger and frustration at the universe or the God of your understanding. But even that doesn't bring you relief. Where can you turn for comfort and healing (if not cure)? How do you live a good life under these conditions?

If you have experienced any of these feelings, you are experiencing the classic process of grieving, as defined by psychologist Elisabeth Kübler-Ross, author of the groundbreaking book *On Death and Dying* (1969). First, there is *anger,* which brings the blame. Then you *deny* that it's really happening, except that it is, so you start *bargaining* with the God of your understanding. When none of those do the trick, you slip into *depression.* From that darkness emerges the first stage in healing: *acceptance.*

We show you how you can use the Intuitive Arts to cycle through the stages of grief to reach the enlightenment and acceptance of peace. To begin, you map out the next 12 months as an astrological year using an ephemeris to note which planets are in a transiting retrograde and for how long. Remember retrogrades ℞ from Chapter 6? Now we put them to practical use. There are many sources to find an accurate ephemeris on the Internet, but one we found is at www.astrology.com/retrograde.html.

We have five cards to play: anger, denial, bargaining, depression, and acceptance. As you shuffle your Tarot deck, meditate on these concepts, using your Psychic Intuition to envision the year that lies before you. You are seeking to know how and when to progress through each stage in the cycle of grief. We have selected five cards to illustrate each stage:

Anger	5 of Wands
Denial	7 of Cups
Bargaining	The Devil
Depression	9 of Swords
Acceptance	Temperance

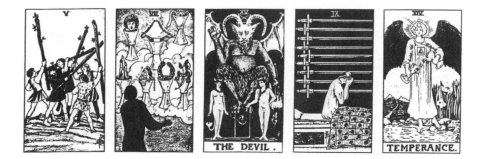

From left, these cards serve as symbols for the phases of grieving: 5 of Wands, anger; 7 of Cups, denial; the Devil, bargaining; 9 of Swords, depression; and Temperance, acceptance.

We offer these to use as a visualization before you do your own Five-Card Spread, asking this request of the Tarot, *"Show me how I must navigate the stages of grieving my illness or disability."*

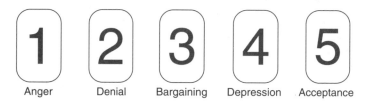

1	2	3	4	5
Anger	Denial	Bargaining	Depression	Acceptance

This Five-Card Spread Tarot reading can be used in conjunction with an astrological map of the year's transiting retrogrades ℞ to gain insight into your path through grieving.

Compare your Tarot reading to your astrological map of transiting retrogrades for the next 12 months. Where does the Tarot card for each grieving stage fall on your astrological map? For example, if the bargaining card in your reading is the 2 of Cups and it falls on the calendar during a Venus ♀ retrograde, this signals a strong positive time to surrender to the healing power of redefining your relationship—to yourself, to your condition, to your loved ones and others around you, to the God of your understanding. Use your Psychic Intuition to link the Tarot reading and the transiting astrological retrogrades to gain insight into which direction the energy of the universe will be heading as you are working through each stage of grief and chart its unique course.

A variation on this exercise is to ask follow-up questions as you go. For instance, when the depression card in your Five-Card Spread is revealed, you may want to ask, *"How long will this grieving stage last?"* Turn up another card, setting it just above the depression card. Then you may want to ask, *"What are my resources and support as I deal with this stage?"* Turn up another card, setting it just below the depression card. Take some time to make notes on your reading, noting how the energy of a particular astrological retrograde might influence each stage or ideas about bolstering your support network during each stage as you move toward acceptance and the healing that accompanies it.

Redirecting Your Efforts: From Tarot's Death to Tarot's Magician

Oh no, not the Death card! This is the card behind all of our fears as we face health problems. But let's take a closer look at the imagery of this card. It's the card about the power of regeneration, and it can give us clues to how to find new energy and new beginnings. It can be the beginning of transformation.

In this card, Death appears as a skeleton riding a white horse toward a humble and beseeching priest, the symbol of spiritual advice; a woman looks away from Death, and a child holds Death's gaze. Beneath Death is the fallen king, whose crown rolls on the ground. Remember how the Tower blows the crown off the king's castle? Death carries the banner of life unfurling a five-petal rose, which evokes the imagery of the thousand-petal lotus chakra of enlightenment. Even though death and destruction lie at the horse's feet, the Sun rises, promising hope.

This powerful card heralds transformation and rejuvenation—a dramatic change in your life. For one thing to live, another must die. The lesson of this card—which is associated with the astrological sign of Scorpio ♏—is that your path to transformative healing is not in putting old things on simmer or merely stashing them on the shelf. You really *do* have to release old energies and karma that are no longer of use to you and let them pass away. This might be painful because those things might have brought you happiness in the past. But it is only through the death of old beliefs and old practices that new ways of being are birthed. Take some time to meditate upon Tarot's Death card and write in your Intuitive Arts notebook about what must come to an end, what must "die" in your life.

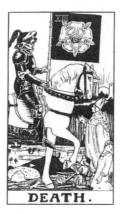

Tarot's Death card is the card of evolution and metamorphosis.

Chances are, you already have a glimpse of your new life ahead. One ceremony often practiced in the Unity Church is that of the burning bowl. We will call this the regeneration burning bowl ceremony. (Remember from Chapter 3 the healing process of the Fire Element? To prepare a burning bowl, place sand in the bottom of a fireproof dish. Put the dish on a safe surface, such as a table or in front of your fireplace. Fire becomes air; the ashes become earth?) From the notes you made in meditation on Tarot's Death card, write statements on strips of paper of things that are bringing you pain. They may be things directly surrounding your illness, such as "pain," "fatigue," or "depression." Or they could be about the frustrating challenges of your illness: "hassling with insurance paperwork," "expensive medications," "going back for *another* treatment," "family members who don't listen," or "too many physical limitations." Or they could be about the inner work you have been doing surrounding your feelings about your condition or situation, such as "unforgiveness," "indulgences," "my fractious relationship with my spouse," "my body image," or "the disapproving messages from my father." You will light these on fire and drop them on the sand in your burning bowl, watching as they burn one by one. As you do, say out loud, "I release the energy of ...."

Now, get up, grab your bowl of ashes and your car keys, and go to a place that is *your* place—a place where you can find peace, a place that inspires you and calms you. Don't worry; we'll be waiting when you come back. When you get there, cast the ashes from your burning bowl to the wind. If you feel comfortable saying it out loud, say, *"I am alive. I embrace my life as it is meant to be lived."* You have transformed your personal energy to become Tarot's Magician.

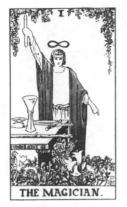

THE MAGICIAN.

The Magician is about unleashing your creative power. It is about new beginnings.

Transformation and Destruction: Pluto ♀ Power

Transformative transiting Pluto ♀ is the catalyst for profoundly powerful change unfolding in our lives from birth to death. Because it takes Pluto 248 years to orbit the Sun, it can spend anywhere from 11 to 32 years in an astrological sign—which is why Pluto is sometimes called the generational planet, as its influence is felt across a generation.

Pluto ♀ moved into Sagittarius ♐ in 1995 and will stay there until 2008. That means Carolyn, whose Sun ☉ sign is Sagittarius, will undergo major transformation during that time. Indeed, already she has lost her father, gotten married, changed jobs, changed homes, given birth to twins, gotten divorced, changed homes again, and turned 40—and there's plenty more time. Pluto has immense power, and its transformation can be overwhelming (yes, Carolyn says)—sometimes physically overwhelming. Pluto has this way of breaking down old ego structures (yes, Carolyn says, I know). Pluto is associated with the mythological lord of the Underworld, the descent into darkness, as well as the regenerative power of Tarot's Death. But Pluto also represents the unconscious mind brought to light.

When Pluto transits over your natal Sun ☉ and Moon ☽, it's another episode of transformation and rebirth. For each of us, the height of Pluto energy is when Pluto swings around to square your natal Pluto ♀ □ ♀—roughly sometime between the ages of 36 and 48. For many of us, this is when we start asking life's tough questions. It's when we start becoming sharply aware of our own mortality. We may make some illogical choices. Pluto knows that—and knows that transformation isn't always neat and clean. Transformation can be marked by grief, despair, a little madness. But beyond the darkness, if we surrender to it, is resurrection. Surrender acknowledges there is only so much control you have over the course of your disease or illness. When you get to the point of surrender—the Hanged Man—you can unleash the creative power of the Magician.

How Pluto transits the angles of your astrological birth chart reveals powerful insights into the turning points of your life. If you'll remember that the angular houses—the 1st house of body and self, the 4th house of home and family, the 7th house of marriage and partnerships, and the 10th house of career and community leadership—are the health houses, it only makes sense that each life juncture is a turning point in your health.

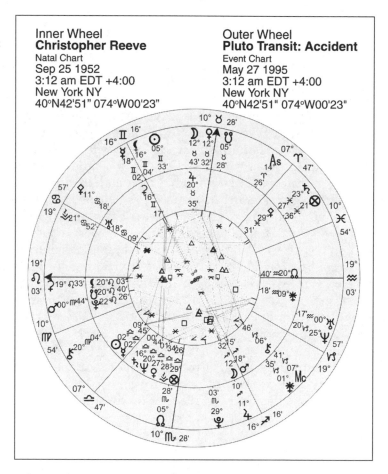

Inner Wheel
Christopher Reeve
Natal Chart
Sep 25 1952
3:12 am EDT +4:00
New York NY
40°N42'51" 074°W00'23"

Outer Wheel
Pluto Transit: Accident
Event Chart
May 27 1995
3:12 am EDT +4:00
New York NY
40°N42'51" 074°W00'23"

Christopher Reeve's Pluto ♀ transit.

Let's take a look at what was going on with Pluto on the date of Christopher Reeve's horseback-riding accident. In this chart, the outer wheel is the date of the accident, while the inner wheel is his birth chart. Sure enough, transiting Pluto shows up in Scorpio ♏ in Reeve's 4th house of home and family. Scorpio is the sign of regeneration, of letting go of one life (invincible physical strength) and rebirthing a new life (voice of courage). Reeve's natal Pluto in his 1st house often means a powerful person who has the ability to influence the public. This is a person with a strong personal identity who communicates his beliefs with great conviction. One of the most admirable qualities of Reeve, post-accident, has been his strong commitment to making others understand disability compassionately.

Healing Peace

In this chapter, we have guided you through making the decision to grow with the opportunity your disease or illness has presented you. Along the way, we have shown you how the Intuitive Arts can direct you to embrace acceptance, and the peace that can bring. If you can find the beauty in your health challenges, you will heal your body, heal your relationships, and heal your soul.

chapter 8

Infinite Choices: Well-Being Through Eternity

Choose again: Reincarnation and second chances
Forgiveness and redemption
12 Karma Street: The house of life lessons
Rising above: Completing life's assignment
The road less traveled: Nodal pairs
Meeting life's challenge: The World
Chiron ⚷: The Wounded Healer
Ceres ⚳: Your astrological legacy
Star and Moon meditation

Every moment is a choice—a choice to move toward the infinite wisdom of the God of your understanding, or to shrink away in fear or confusion. It's a choice to breathe in the vitality and success of Tarot's World card, or to delight in life's mysteries revealed in the Tower card—or flee, forgetting we are on fire. These moment-by-moment choices add up to the infinite choices of a life lived, its meaning, and your well-being through eternity. In this chapter, we use Astrology, Tarot, and Psychic Intuition to heed the beckoning call of eternity's deep mysteries. We use the Tarot to guide you through forgiveness and embracing life's second chances and Astrology to guide you through your karmic life lessons. Along the way, we meet the asteroid Ceres and the planetoid Chiron, who can give you messages about healing your wounds and leaving your legacy.

Choose Again: Reincarnation and Second Chances

In the movie *Groundhog Day*, Bill Murray plays a television journalist assigned to report on Punxsutawney Phil's big day, February 2. Along the way, Andie McDowell catches his eye, and he is in hot pursuit. Only he just has it all wrong. He's a major turnoff, a bumbling insensitive boob, and she keeps rejecting him. But each day, the alarm goes off, and Murray's character wakes up to the same day—Groundhog Day—and gets a chance to try again. Progress is slow, but each time he is a little wiser.

We love this movie because it's all about getting the chance to keep at it until we get it right. "Choose again," is the familiar phrase from the spiritual teachings of A Course in Miracles (a unique self-study spiritual thought system that teaches love and inner peace)—meaning that every moment offers you the chance to choose differently, to choose better. You may be able to look back on your life and see some choices you made about your health that you would do oh so differently now. There is a promise of redemption proffered in a second chance. How many of us have said, "If I had this life to do over again ...." The branches of the Intuitive Arts don't always assume a belief in reincarnation. For the most part, this is left to the individual. So while you might not believe in reincarnation, you probably do believe in second chances.

Groundhog Day is a fitting metaphor for second chances. It is almost Groundhog Day as we write this chapter. The Sun ☉ has just moved into Aquarius ♒, and the first tiny buds are sprouting from the cottonwoods. Aquarius represents the dawning of a new age, a bright promise of a world free from the darkness of the past. In the Tarot, the Tower card is connected to Aquarius, for the bolt from the blue is the catalyst for true inventiveness. The Star card, too, is connected to Aquarius, the dreamer of impossible dreams. The Star signifies humanitarian efforts and the virtues of hope, faith, and charity. It is a universal sign of hope for a better tomorrow. Certainly, the groundhog is looking for a better tomorrow—the first sign of spring. Ever hopeful, he pokes his head out at midwinter, hoping for no shadow.

Whatever your personal beliefs about God and an afterlife, you probably do believe in the eternal. There are as many ways to describe it as there are spiritual paths—Heaven, the afterlife, nirvana, a state of bliss, the spirit world. Whatever you believe, you probably do believe you will leave a spiritual and emotional legacy long after your body turns to dust. In this chapter, we use Astrology, Tarot, and Psychic Intuition to guide you in revealing the choices of the infinite.

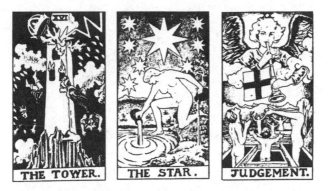

Tarot's Tower is the catalyst, the Star is the dreamer of impossible dreams, and Judgement signals your great awakening.

Pull out the Judgement card from your Tarot deck. This card represents the big cosmic wake-up call—the one Bill Murray so desperately needed in *Groundhog Day* that time stood still until he got it. In this card, the angel blows the trumpet. Souls arise to a greater purpose. This is the card of self-actualization, and it can come up often when you are seeking earnestly to improve on your health and spiritual well-being. It signals your great awakening.

Forgiveness and Redemption

If you could erase some of the mistakes you have made in the way you treat your body, yourself, and others, would you? Forgiveness and redemption won't give you the pink lungs of a baby again if you have smoked most of your life, but it can give you the peace of mind that gives you your best chance at physical and spiritual health for now and beyond.

Along with reincarnation comes the belief in past lives. Again, the interpretation is up to you. If you don't really believe in past lives, you probably do understand the influence of your genes or family background, your childhood, and psychological "baggage." You probably can see patterns of behavior in your family background that need to be worked out. Maybe you can get your mind around life lessons and evolutionary paths. And if you have ever been hurt and it took you a long time to get over it, you understand the pain and power of forgiveness.

In these two exercises, we use aromatherapy, the Tarot, and the chakras to help your Psychic Intuition guide you in forgiveness. The aromatherapy blends and affirmations are used with the kind permission of Francoise Rapp, an aromatherapist and alchemist trained in her native France and based in San Diego (www.aromalchemy.com).

Forgive Yourself

To create a custom aromatherapy blend, combine the following essential oils:

- 3 drops rose otto
- 8 drops sandalwood
- 5 drops geranium
- 4 drops sage

Add the essential oils to a 10-ounce bottle, using organic vegetable oil to fill. Prepare a warm bath. Sit quietly for a few moments before entering the water. Close your eyes and take a few deep breaths. Now, open your eyes. As you meditate on the Queen of Cups, anoint your heart chakra and solar plexus. You are opening your heart and summoning your power.

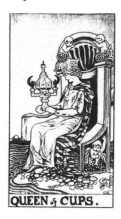

Inspire your heart chakra with the cup of self-forgiveness and healing energy.

Pour a few drops into your warm bath water and soak for at least 15 minutes. Pour a few drops into the palms of your hands and inhale deeply. Repeat this affirmation three times: *I release any and all negative or unhealthy attitudes toward myself. I forgive myself and ask for healing.*

Forgive Others

For this blend, combine the following essential oils:

- ☯ 3 drops rose otto
- ☯ 6 drops sandalwood
- ☯ 3 drops German chamomile
- ☯ 5 drops frankincense

As you meditate on the Knight of Cups riding to extend the cup of forgiveness, anoint your heart chakra, solar plexus, and third eye.

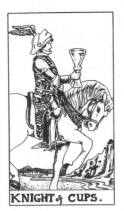

Inspire your heart chakra by extending the cup of forgiveness and healing energy to those you love.

Pour a few drops into your warm bath water and soak for at least 15 minutes. Pour a few drops into the palms of your hands and inhale deeply. Use this affirmation: *I understand you. I accept and love you for who you are. I forgive you.*

12 Karma Street: The House of Life Lessons

Think of your karmic life lessons as buried treasure. Your astrological birth chart is the map, and the "x" is on the 12th house. The 12th house is the point at which the self—the 1st house—has completed its journey and meets the soul, where body meets the spirit. Successfully navigating the 1st through 11th houses leads you to the doorstep of the 12th house, the place where you can transcend life's trials and tribulations.

By looking at which planets reside in your 12th house, you can unlock its karmic treasure chest. What's inside can free you from destructive life patterns. This house offers a true challenge. Those who encounter the challenge of the 12th house before they are ready might not be able to handle it well and might turn to self-destructive behaviors. The 12th house can lift you to a higher consciousness—or it can be your undoing.

The Sun ☉. Your need for privacy and introspection is vital to maintaining balance between your inner life and the active daily routines of work and home. You were born with an obligation to serve others, but you prefer to do it from behind the scenes. Your mission is to find truths that ring for all humankind.

The Moon ☽. You have a strong intuitive sense of others' emotions, but you may be easily stung by others' insensitivity. This might keep you in self-protective mode, and you may need to process your emotions slowly, through meditation or exploring spiritual traditions. Your challenge is to do this in a positive way. The Moon in the 12th house means your emotions find their source in your subconscious and/or in past life experiences.

Mercury ☿. You think a lot about everything, and sometimes you keep your emotions to yourself. Your decisions are often intuitive and your mental process is influenced by childhood memories, your subconscious, or past lives. Your challenge is to resist the lure of "mind escape," staying in the here and now. It's a challenge to keep your mind from trailing off into the ether. With a healthy dose of reality, Mercury in the 12th house can be highly intelligent, futuristic, and headstrong. You may be hard to read because you "incubate" your ideas before you speak your truth.

Venus ♀. You feel deeply and compassionately, approaching life through art and creativity, and you are happy to serve the community with your insights. You may be devoted to exploring divine wisdom. You relish delving into the heart of a matter and have an uncanny knack for uncovering mysteries about yourself or others. Creativity is so pronounced in a 12th house Venus that we would say you are *obligated* to create. The deeper you go into your creative side, the more you will hone your intuition.

Mars ♂. You have the passionate emotions, thoughts, and feelings of a warrior, but you may find them too perplexing to examine—and just as fiercely as you feel them, you may keep them under wraps. Your emotions are connected to past lives, childhood memories, or your unconscious mind. Your challenge is that if you are pushed to your limits, your suppressed anger rears its ugly head—and you strike back with a fury that surprises no one and everyone—including *you!* Your duty is to harness your fierceness to focus it on achieving change for the greater good—your karmic destiny and the world's.

Jupiter ♃. You possess faith and a philosophical personality. Some call a 12th house Jupiter the "angel on your shoulder." With Jupiter in the 12th house, you seem protected from above. You may be drawn to a spiritual tradition. Your challenge is to avoid embracing fanaticism in overdevotion or allowing your passions to express themselves too expansively, or with narcissism.

Saturn ♄. Often a loner, you play by the rules and respect boundaries—sometimes to a fault! Your challenge is that you may isolate yourself, leaving yourself without a confidant to share life's experiences. You may consider yourself unworthy or unequal to the task life sets before you, and you may worry any time you perceive a lack of structure in your life. These fears are linked to your past lives, childhood memories, or subconscious, and it's your challenge to transcend them and embrace the Zen of organizing Saturn at its most creative and intrepid.

Uranus ♅. Uranus wants you to embrace your *own* path, whatever that may be—nonconforming, dancing to your own beat. In the 12th house, though, fear may overtake you, so have courage! You are an innovative thinker who delights in finding the "new" way, and are drawn to the enigmatic. You will want your life's work to be unusual. Your challenge is that you will feel so far "out there" you may have trouble finding company among your more ordinary peers. You must look at your past influences to unlock the key to your deeper understanding.

Neptune ♆. Neptune is the planet of dreams and you are a dreamer with deep psychic knowing. You may be artistic, musical, poetic, psychic, spiritual—or all of the above. Your intuition reaches deep into your own body, mind, and spirit, and, perhaps, also into the collective consciousness of all humanity. Your challenge is that a search for spiritual meaning is vital. Early in life, if the path is strewn with too many conventional messages, you may feel isolated. You will want to protect yourself from negative energy, and move toward situations that are peaceful and positive.

Pluto ♇. You have the ability to infuse your life with spiritual knowing. Your deepest dream is to unite with the God of your understanding—to touch the divine. Your task is to remove any

163

obstacles in your path. This is quite a challenge—it means dissolving the self formed in the 1st house. Your lesson is faith—to take the leap into the unknown, to believe in what you cannot yet see.

If you have no planets in the 12th house, does it mean you have no hidden desires? Well, that would be no fun! We all have some element of mystery about us, so if you don't have planets in the 12th house, it may mean a little more detective work is needed to find the clues to your hidden issues. Start by finding the sign on the 12th house cusp. What planet rules that astrological sign? Your hidden desires may be focused on the house where that planet resides. For instance, say you have an empty 12th house but Pisces ♓ is on the cusp. Pisces is ruled by Neptune ♆, and Neptune falls in your 4th house, the house of family. You may have idealized your family or neglected to see family issues for what they really are, and this may be diminishing your health. Your 12th house challenge is to look at these issues, drawing upon your dreams, Psychic Intuition, and spiritual practice.

Rising: Completing Life's Assignment

Your rising sign represents more than the persona you present to others. It is the person you are becoming. For clues into your life assignments, we look to your ascendant. We compiled a chart of ascendants of some famous people, along with their life assignments. Take note of the special blossoming potential that your ascendant indicates for you. Make these areas of your life healthy and positive. Devote your attention to cultivating them, and you may find the obstacles to your eternal wellness are not so overwhelming.

For example, perhaps you are considered frail by others, but you are an Aries ♈ ascendant; it may be that you are called to cultivate independence. If you look back on the areas in which you have struggled in life, you will likely find such challenges have come your way. A Cancer ♋ ascendant needs a strong family foundation to thrive; if you lack nurturing relationships around you, your health will suffer, and your challenge is to learn those nurturing skills.

Ascendant	Blossoming Potential For ...	Celebrity(s)	Her/His Mission
Aries ♈	Independence	Bette Midler *Sagittarius ♐ with Aries ♈ rising*	To engender enthusiasm in others; to push the envelope.

Ascendant	Blossoming Potential For ...	Celebrity(s)	Her/His Mission
Taurus ♉	Infusing the material with spirit	George Lucas *Taurus ♉ with Taurus ♉ rising*	To use art to inspire others' creativity.
Gemini ♊	Honest, emotional storytelling	Bruce Springsteen *Libra ♎ with Gemini ♊ rising*	To communicate to others the importance of seeking and speaking the truth; planting seeds of thought.
Cancer ♋	Parenting a loving, nurturing family or creative life	Stephen King *Virgo ♍ with Cancer ♋ rising*	To evoke emotion; to nurture the psyche and explore the depth of human emotion.
Leo ♌	Nurturing self-love, self-respect, and self-confidence	Hilary Rodham Clinton *Scorpio ♏ with Leo ♌ rising* Maya Angelou *Aries ♈ with Leo ♌ rising* Christopher Reeve *Libra ♎ with Leo ♌ rising*	To learn not to be so hard on herself/himself; to understand that her/his emotional needs are at odds with the way she/he presents her/himself; complete self-acceptance; learn not to discount emotional needs.
Virgo ♍	Touching the divine nature of the universe and its sacred patterns	Madonna *Leo ♌ with Virgo ♍ rising* Oprah Winfrey *Aquarius ♒ with Virgo ♍ rising*	To become more focused, more spiritual, more discerning, and self-affirming; to experience their work as sacred.
Libra ♎	Facilitating relationships and fostering equity	The Dalai Lama *Cancer ♋ with Libra ♎ rising*	To become a natural diplomat, tolerant, fair, always ready to

Ascendant	Blossoming Potential For ...	Celebrity(s)	Her/His Mission
			listen to different viewpoints. A Libra rising has a high desire for others to feel in harmony when they come into his/her physical presence.
Scorpio ♏	Influence through charisma	Katharine Hepburn *Taurus ♉ with Scorpio ♏ rising*	To cultivate high intuition about others' unspoken feelings and motivations; to overcome caution and suspicion at outset of a relationship.
Sagittarius ♐	Traveling to infinity and beyond!	Princess Diana *Cancer ♋ with Sagittarius ♐ rising*	To encourage others to think in a different way; to break through old conditioning, and shed fears.
Capricorn ♑	Responsible caregiving	Sean Connery *Virgo ♍ with Capricorn ♑ rising*	To focus on productivity, material gain, resourcefulness.
Aquarius ♒	Crystal revelations	Michael J. Fox *Gemini ♊ with Aquarius ♒ rising*	To advocate change and human advancement. Aquarius rising is extremely aware of how we are all connected. They have a high awareness of the social and global implications of personal actions and a genuine interest in the good of the whole over personal welfare.

Ascendant	Blossoming Potential For ...	Celebrity(s)	Her/His Mission
Pisces ♓	Loving unconditionally, without loss of self	Robert Redford Leo ♌ *with Pisces ♓ rising*	To challenge old principles if they are not good for the group consciousness; to take on humanitarian causes.

The Road Less Traveled: Nodal Pairs ☊ ☋

The Moon's Nodes in your astrological birth chart are karmic touchstones. The South Node ☋ represents the lessons you have already mastered, past life lessons, while the North Node ☊ points to the lessons you are here to learn in this life. You are no doubt already getting cosmic feedback about these two paths. The lessons of the South Node are easily incorporated into this life's successes. But take on the challenge of the North Node and you stand ready to evolve in new and exciting ways that redefine who you are and lead to your optimal health and well-being.

The Nodes appear opposite each other in your astrological birth chart.

North Node ☊ In ...	South Node ☋ In ...	Karmic Lessons Learned, Lessons to Master
Aries ♈	Libra ♎	☋ **Already learned:** Cooperation, dependence ☊ **Need to learn:** Independence, initiative, self-confidence **Challenge:** Use relationship skills to build leadership skills
Taurus ♉	Scorpio ♏	☋ **Already learned:** Charisma, regeneration, transformation ☊ **Need to learn:** Security, new map of the world **Challenge:** Infuse the material with spiritual beauty and power

North Node ☊ In ...	South Node ☋ In ...	Karmic Lessons Learned, Lessons to Master
Gemini ♊	Sagittarius ♐	☋ **Already learned:** Adventuring, honesty ☊ **Need to learn:** Communication, seeing both sides of a problem **Challenge:** Channel your truth quest into constructive communication
Cancer ♋	Capricorn ♑	☋ **Already learned:** Goal setting and attainment, success ☊ **Need to learn:** Sensitivity, nurturing **Challenge:** Derive sense of achievement through sharing emotions, caregiving
Leo ♌	Aquarius ♒	☋ **Already learned:** About changing the world for the good of all ☊ **Need to learn:** Big-hearted openness **Challenge:** Broaden noble love for humanity, make heartfelt connections, become altruistic
Virgo ♍	Pisces ♓	☋ **Already learned:** Compassion, intuition ☊ **Need to learn:** Sacred service, meticulous organization **Challenge:** Tell your personal story to help others
Libra ♎	Aries ♈	☋ **Already learned:** Independence, self-confidence, initiative ☊ **Need to learn:** Balance, harmony **Challenge:** Balance self with other(s), learn to nurture group or community achievement
Scorpio ♏	Taurus ♉	☋ **Already learned:** Building a solid, stable life ☊ **Need to learn:** Transforming change, letting go **Challenge:** The power of metamorphosis

North Node ☊ In …	South Node ☋ In …	Karmic Lessons Learned, Lessons to Master
Sagittarius ♐	Gemini ♊	☋ **Already learned:** Lightning thought, processing multiple viewpoints
		☊ **Need to learn:** Cutting to the truth, seeking greater truth
		Challenge: Become a divine adventurer
Capricorn ♑	Cancer ♋	☋ **Already learned:** How to parent in a loving, nurturing, creative way
		☊ **Need to learn:** Responsible behavior, planning and goal setting
		Challenge: Bring caring touch to positions of responsibility, requiring wisdom
Aquarius ♒	Leo ♌	☋ **Already learned:** Expansive and generous nature
		☊ **Need to learn:** Humanitarianism
		Challenge: Look beyond the self to use generosity to create community good
Pisces ♓	Virgo ♍	☋ **Already learned:** Sacred duty, attention to detail
		☊ **Need to learn:** intuition, deep knowing, compassion
		Challenge: Connect sacred duty and intuition to achieve profound understanding of humanity and the divine

How do you know when you have arrived, when the quest to become what you *will* become has been reached, and you can rest in contentment? Here is where Tarot's World card comes in, the card of self-actualization and attainment. The World promises fulfillment of all your most heartfelt desires. Now you have a deep and abiding understanding of your karmic gifts and lessons. The World sends you the message that you now have the freedom to move ahead and pursue deeper growth: enlightenment. Take a few moments to visualize what attainment might look and feel like to you.

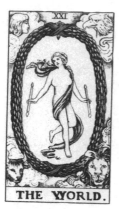

THE WORLD.

With Tarot's World, you have understood your karmic lessons and will manifest your best self.

Chiron ⚷: The Wounded Healer

Chiron ⚷ is a planetoid orbiting the outer realm of our solar system, and he is often called the Wounded Healer. This celestial body takes his name from a centaur (half-man, half-horse) in Greek mythology who, after his parents abandoned him, healed and matured into a wise and compassionate healer and teacher. The lesson of Chiron is that overcoming our greatest emotional burden can be a great source of healing wisdom for ourselves and others. Look for Chiron ⚷ in your astrological birth chart. Knowing in which astrological house Chiron appears tells us in which area you must act. Turn to Appendix A for a review of the houses and their areas of importance in our lives.

Chiron in Aries ⚷ ♈. *Your wound: Sense of self.* You may have inflicted so much pain on yourself that you find it difficult to achieve peace with yourself. You may wallow in self-pity and punish yourself for what you are not. Embrace and accept yourself as you are. Celebrate your strengths and reach out to others who are experiencing similar pain. Give your time to causes helping others with self-esteem and appearance issues, such as eating disorders.

Chiron in Taurus ⚷ ♉. *Your wound: Neglect, deprivation.* What you have is never enough. It may come from your childhood, in which your parents withheld affection or you competed with siblings for attention. You may have experienced monetary or material deprivation. You have a deep yearning for security and the delight of sensual pleasures such as food, physical affection, and pampering. Still, it's unsatisfying. You must learn to cherish what you have. Give your time to causes that help others who have experienced lack of plenty, such as homeless or neglected children.

Chiron in Gemini ⚷ ♊. *Your wound: Self-doubt.* You doubt your intellect and your instincts, and your greatest fear is that others will not understand you. You may exhaustively seek knowledge. Instead, congratulate yourself on what you do know. Learn to listen to your instincts and note your successes when you act on them. Put yourself in situations where you can teach others a unique skill that you know well, and it will build your confidence. Give your time to causes dealing with learning disorders or illiteracy.

Chiron in Cancer ⚷ ♋. *Your wound: Neglecting your own pain.* You feel unworthy of love, and you turn your energy outward, giving too much to others. You have a strong desire to nurture, but you give it all away, and sometimes people take advantage of you. Your Chiron call is to give love to yourself and open yourself to letting others love you. Once you do, you can start giving again in a more balanced way.

Chiron in Leo ⚷ ♌. *Your wound: Stifled expression.* You want to be adored, but you feel you have never been given the chance to let your light shine. You want to be in the spotlight, and you desire to be flooded with compliments. When others aren't as effusive as you want them to be about your many talents, you are quick to retreat in wounded frustration. Chiron invites you to reassess your vision, to stop those *Tonight Show* fantasies and instead express the talents you already possess in the arenas that are being presented to you right here, right now.

Chiron in Virgo ⚷ ♍. *Your wound: Imperfection.* You believe you will never measure up. You can only see your faults and can fall into bemoaning them. Your fear is that the devil is in the details, and some unattended detail will send your endeavor careening out of control. This makes you very controlling or may hold you back from embarking on any endeavor for fear it will be imperfect. Chiron in Virgo encourages you to look at how your imperfections and those of others move you to healing. Relax: You are not perfect and you can learn from it, Chiron says.

Chiron in Libra ⚷ ♎. *Your wound: Dependence and idealism in love.* You have a fear of losing your love at the same time you fear that the relationship doesn't meet your ideals. You may cling to people to the point of breaking your spirit, losing sight of whether the relationship even works for you. You may subconsciously sabotage relationships that fail to live up to your standards. You shy away from conflict, but you are not aware of your own inner conflict when you expect so much from your relationships. Chiron in Libra compels you to embrace conflict and understand that it can guide you to greater intimacy. By growing comfortable with disagreeing with people, you can learn to let go of those people you should let go of and bridge the gap with those who are different from you but entirely worth it. Your social causes are relationship counseling or codependent support groups.

Chiron in Scorpio ⚷ ♏. *Your wound: Fear of losing what you have.* You live in utter dread of losing your most vital self—your life, your possessions, your loved ones, your home, your soul. You believe you can never retrieve what you might lose, and you hang on to it dearly. At its worst, a Chiron wound in Scorpio can lead to dominance, jealousy, and emotional stinginess. Your Chiron lesson is to learn what loss can teach you about living and healing. When you learn this, you can open your wound to the world and have a powerful capacity to teach others about the role of pain in healing. You may find your social causes are in bereavement counseling or stress management.

Chiron in Sagittarius ⚷ ♐. *Your wound: Fear of being confined.* You believe you were meant to live a life of adventure and achieve great wisdom. You are programmed for risk taking and you can be restless, but something is holding you back. You feel you are not living out the adventurous life you desire. You need to be free and explore new ideas and meet new people, but you feel imprisoned in a mundane life. Your task is to see your place in the world. You must acknowledge the power of your expansive nature yet see the opportunities that are rooted in your daily life.

Chiron in Capricorn ⚷ ♑. *Your wound: Fear of not being recognized.* You are working hard—harder than anyone—yet you are not achieving the status and respect you believe you deserve. You are ambitious, and you can often get so caught up in your vision of the higher goal that you don't take time to stop and assess your accomplishments. Cast aside your need for validation for your success and instead acknowledge your own value. Taking stock of what you have achieved will provide you with the self-satisfaction you seek. You will find your social causes in helping others realize their potential, such as in career counseling.

Chiron in Aquarius ⚷ ♒. *Your wound: Alienation.* No matter how much you try, you feel so different from everyone else that you feel isolated. You are deeply seeking a sense of belonging to a group or a larger humanitarian cause. You may be exacerbating your sense of alienation by being aloof. Your challenge is not to pull away or pretend to be someone you're not. Chiron invites you to be yourself and let yourself be a little eccentric. Give your time to groups that support individual expression or champion human rights.

Chiron in Pisces ⚷ ♓. *Your wound: Losing your faith.* At some time in life, you were betrayed, and you may have become bitter. Your heart is closed, and you want to avoid any pain of future disappointment. Yet, you still have a deep desire to understand human motivations and the sacred patterns of the universe. Your disillusionment and feelings of betrayal are holding you back from understanding your connection to the universe. Your Chiron challenge is to not turn your back on your beliefs, but transcend. Understand that everything happens for a reason. Suffering leads to great beauty. Questioning your faith and core beliefs can enrich and deepen them. Give your time to causes that nourish individuals seeking their higher purpose or are helping others reconnect to the spiritual path.

Progressions: Evolution in Progress

Astrology offers an easy way to check your progress on the path of personal growth. It's called the progressed chart, which is different from a transit chart. A transit chart captures what was going on with the planets for everyone at a specific moment in time—a slice of life. But a progressed chart is one that advances the planets forward from *your* birth chart.

Let's look at Bruce Springsteen's progressed chart on the date his Grammy Award–winning CD *The Rising* was released. In this chart, the outer wheel is Bruce's progressed chart, the inner wheel his birth chart. When we analyze a progressed chart, some of the things we look at are changes in signs or houses, planets that go retrograde or direct, or a planetary movement that changes an aspect.

On the day of the release of *The Rising*, Bruce's progressed Moon ☽ had just begun making a positive, lucky connection with his natal Jupiter ♃ in Capricorn ♑, in the form of a trine △. This points to financial success and renewed creativity. His progressed Moon was in his 4th house, coming into a conjunction with his natal Sun ☉ in Libra ♎. This indicates he would create music that would reveal his own personal evolution and represent a homecoming.

The progressed Sun has moved into Scorpio ♏, which connects in the form of a sextile ✶ to natal Jupiter in Capricorn. This indicates Bruce would tap into new, powerful ways to transform others, and the arena would be his 8th house, the house of new resources and new energy. *The Rising* was notable as the recording reunion of the E Street Band. After more than a decade off, the E Street Band proved better than ever—definitely providing new resources for the Boss!

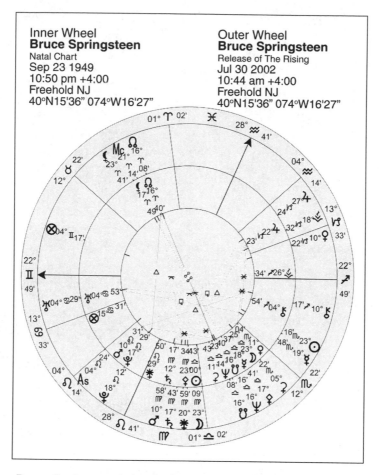

Inner Wheel
Bruce Springsteen
Natal Chart
Sep 23 1949
10:50 pm +4:00
Freehold NJ
40°N15'36" 074°W16'27"

Outer Wheel
Bruce Springsteen
Release of The Rising
Jul 30 2002
10:44 am +4:00
Freehold NJ
40°N15'36" 074°W16'27"

Bruce Springsteen's birth chart, progressed to the release date of his CD The Rising.

The Asteroids: Nurturing Your Legacy

Chiron isn't the only asteroid that has a pull on you and your potential legacy. We'd like to introduce you to a few more. Ceres ⚳, Juno ⚵, Pallas Athene ⚴, and Vesta ⚶ are asteroids named after Greek goddesses, and they bring a goddess touch to your birth chart.

Asteroid	Realm	Influences
Ceres ⚳	Motherhood	Parenting, nurturing, natural cycles, fertility
Juno ⚵	Marriage	Partnerships, control
Pallas Athene ⚴	Wisdom	Intelligence; physical strength and agility; understanding; psychological healing
Vesta ⚶	Power	Fulfillment, service, power

For this chapter, we want to take a closer look at Ceres, the Green goddess of mothering, nurturing, fertility, and agriculture. Ceres ⚳ is the asteroid most often used to gain insight into your style for mothering. But we're going to look at mothering in a more sacred, spiritual—and gender-free—way. When we talk about a legacy, we can talk about it in nurturing terms—mothering or fathering. Who (or what) have you given birth to in your life? How have you nurtured it? What have you not nourished in your life but you wish you had?

In Greek mythology, Ceres is the goddess of nature and its cycles. So when we think of our legacy, think of a field. What have you sown, and what have you reaped? In Astrology, the asteroid Ceres ⚳ is naturally associated with Cancer ♋, the most nurturing sign in the Zodiac, and it is ruled by the Moon ☽, which influences the natural cycles of life. In the Tarot, she connects with the Moon card, which represents intuition.

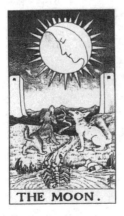

The Moon represents the asteroid Ceres ⚳.

Ceres in Aries ⚳ ♈. Your way of nurturing people is to get out there and fight for them. You are likely to take on so much you are not at peace with yourself. You are the kind of person others call upon when they really need help.

Ceres in Taurus ? ♉. You have built safe structures for those around you. You have an unwavering self-love that is based on the strong and secure foundation you have built for your life. You have brought many others security and beautiful material things that enrich their lives. You grow when supported by sensuality and loyalty.

Ceres in Gemini ? ♊. You are like a butterfly, nurturing the thoughts and ideas of those around you. You are a fresh breeze that plants in others the seeds of new life and new ideas. You thrive when you are learning.

Ceres in Cancer ? ♋. The powerful combination of Ceres and Cancer means that you define the very essence of love, compassion, and nurturing. You have the capacity to take on the wounds of others and heal them. In the big picture, you are in tune with the emotional currents of life, and your power to help others is unending. Your love is genuine and eternal.

Ceres in Leo ? ♌. You are the light of the Sun, and your enthusiasm and vitality inspire others. You encourage others to believe in themselves and discover their creativity and their utmost potential. You receive nurturing with grace and ease and radiate it to others.

Ceres in Virgo ? ♍. You are the healing Earth Mother, with a powerful focus on the health, well-being, and spirit of all people, animals, and plants. You possess the ability to self-sacrifice, and you are gracious in your humility. You bring a purity and precision to the way you heal.

Ceres in Libra ? ♎. You are the peace goddess, and bring justice, fairness, and balance to all you take on. You can soothe others with beauty and serenity. You have the ability to heal disharmony and imbalances in your own life and in others' lives.

Ceres in Scorpio ? ♏. You are protective, loyal, and passionate. You have a powerful ability to seek out the darkness and transform it to light. You are a bridge for others to cross their fears, let go, find renewal, and transform.

Ceres in Sagittarius ? ♐. You nurture big dreams and new horizons. You can take on new adventures with grace, and you support others in taking risks, doing it all joyfully and enthusiastically. You want to explore the world and delight in new discoveries.

Ceres in Capricorn ? ♑. You nurture your own highest aspirations and those of others. You are free with the compliments and encouragement. You show others how to meet their goals through discipline, responsibility, and loyalty. You always follow through.

Ceres in Aquarius ? ♒. Your knack for innovation is where your legacy lies. You are one to chase your dreams. You are a natural leader, with power and conviction. You support those you love—even their wildest dreams. Your legacy is the future.

Ceres in Pisces ⚵ ♓. Your legacy is enchantment. You nurture the dreams and imaginations of yourself and others, and have a deep appreciation for the realm of intuition. You love unconditionally, and you nurture universal love and sacrifice. You are nourished by those who support your dreams.

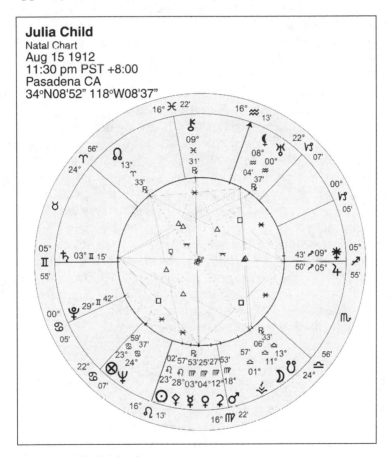

Julia Child's birth chart.

Julia Child is the goddess of the culinary arts in America, so let's see how the asteroid goddesses, as well as the healer Chiron ⚷, influenced her. While her husband was stationed in Paris after World War II, Julia studied at Cordon Bleu. Her Public Broadcasting Service program brought the elegance of French cooking to a public used to a cuisine of potato salad and Jell-O. Julia has a Ceres ⚷ in Earth mother Virgo ♍, and it's in her 4th house of home—a natural pairing for a chef, because we associate nurturing through food. The mutable sign of Virgo is the sign of health and purity. Vesta ⚶ is the goddess who keeps the home fires burning, so with a Vesta in Libra ♎, in her 5th house of entertaining and artistic talent, we know that Julia has a strong need for creating beauty and elegance around her. This proved true despite Julia's growing up a privileged child in Pasadena, California, where the family had a chef in the kitchen. Though cooking skills were not required, Julia was always interested in being the hostess from an early age.

With Juno ⚵ in Sagittarius ♐ in Julia's 7th house of love and marriage, we can see that her style of making a partnership is about discovery. Because her husband loved fine food, as a newlywed and novice cook Julia decided to learn her way about the kitchen. It must have worked; it's said Paul Child adored his wife. Once her first cookbook introducing French cuisine to America took off, he devoted himself to promoting her career. Julia's Chiron ⚷ in Pisces ♓ is in her 10th house of career, indicating she would become known as a singular person with the ability to see beyond traditional views. Julia's Chiron placement tells us she would be a maverick in her chosen career. With Pallas Athene ⚴ in Leo ♌, Julia brings intelligence and strength, courage and enthusiasm to her creative work. Pallas Athene in Leo would bring Julia to a position of educator, with an intelligent approach to food, health, and cooking. In July 2003, master chef Julia Child received the Presidential Medal of Freedom in acknowledgment of her life achievements and contribution to American culinary culture.

Where It All Leads: A Meditation

Take a few deep breaths, get calm, and get your pulse rate down. Now meditate and visualize the way it must have been on the night (or day) you were born. Above you are all the energies of the universe. Spread out above you is all the gentle and ancient wisdom of time. Above you is the choreography of all the movements of your life. Take in a few more deep breaths as you begin to deepen your appreciation for the influences that create your most vital self and chart your most healing path. Take in a deep appreciation for your Creator and the path of your life. Know that every breath is a miracle, every heartbeat an affirmation.

chapter 9

Create Your Most Vital Body, Mind, and Spirit

Vital Signs Portrait: The picture of your health
Intuition rising: A body, mind, and spirit scan
Suit yourself: Tarot Power Portrait
The wild kingdom: Aspects of opportunity and challenge
Emerging patterns: A Tarot analysis
A year of health: Horoscope Spread
Entering the bliss center of health

It is time to put together everything you've learned throughout this book to create a portrait of your most vital body, mind, and spirit. In this chapter, we teach you how to do an Astrology and Tarot body scan that can activate your Psychic Intuition—and invite your most vital self. We also show you how you can do a daily Tarot Power Health Portrait that can show you where your power and resources lie. We pull together all of the Tarot readings you have done for this book so that you can see emerging patterns that may present you challenges in the year ahead. By using a 12-month Horoscope Spread, we coach you in developing a plan for your health in the coming year. And finally, we create a visualization using Tarot, the Buddhist mandala, and the 12 astrological houses that shows you the steps to manifest your highest intentions, dreams, and desires for this life—and beyond.

Vital Signs Portrait

Let's start by pulling together your Vital Signs Portrait. First, look in your astrological birth chart to find in which astrological sign the planets, Nodes, your ascendant, and asteroids appear, and list the placement for each in the following table. Make a few notes here about what you have learned in previous chapters about the influence of each astrological sign on your approach to staying healthy—what do these placements in your birth chart tell you about *your* health? You may want to refer to this table as you do the exercises in this chapter.

Planet	Influences	Astro Sign	Thoughts
Sun ☉	Your self	_____	_____
Moon ☽	Your emotions	_____	_____
Mercury ☿	The way you communicate	_____	_____
Venus ♀	The way you love, forgive	_____	_____
Mars ♂	Your passion, your fire, your anger	_____	_____
Jupiter ♃	Your optimism	_____	_____
Saturn ♄	Your self-discipline	_____	_____
Uranus ♅	Your capacity for change	_____	_____
Neptune ♆	Your compassion, your dreams	_____	_____
Pluto ♇	Your capacity for transformation	_____	_____
North Node ☊	Lessons to learn	_____	_____
South Node ☋	Lessons mastered	_____	_____
Ascendant	What you are becoming	_____	_____
Ceres ⚳	Your legacy	_____	_____
Chiron ⚷	Your wounds to heal	_____	_____

Now, the fun begins. Get out your Tarot deck. For each item in the "Planet" column in the preceding table, choose a card from the Tarot deck—only not at random as with a Tarot reading. Use your Psychic Intuition to select a card that you can return to when you need a portrait of your health. Think of each card as a beacon that illuminates your understanding of your basic constitution, your strengths, and your challenges. As you move through your deck, say "My Sun ☉ sign card," again and again, repeating it like a mantra. Don't think about which card it should be or which card you want it to be. We are trying to turn off your "thinking" mind and tap into your "feeling" mind. Once you have selected a card, lay it face up before you.

One at a time, repeat the exercise for each item, chanting a mantra. List your choices here, and add the astrological signs and houses in which each planet or heavenly body appears.

Planet	Tarot Card	Astro Sign	Astro House
Sun ☉	_____	_____	_____
Moon ☽	_____	_____	_____
Mercury ☿	_____	_____	_____
Venus ♀	_____	_____	_____
Mars ♂	_____	_____	_____
Jupiter ♃	_____	_____	_____
Saturn ♄	_____	_____	_____
Uranus ♅	_____	_____	_____
Neptune ♆	_____	_____	_____
Pluto ♇	_____	_____	_____
North Node ☊	_____	_____	_____
South Node ☋	_____	_____	_____
Ascendant	_____	_____	_____
Ceres ⚳	_____	_____	_____
Chiron ⚷	_____	_____	_____

Now, place each Tarot card literally over your astrological birth chart, laying out each card over the house in which the planet or heavenly body appears. You may want to make a poster-size photocopy of your birth chart for this exercise. A digital photograph of the final result will preserve your Vital Signs Portrait for future reference and insights. Take some time now to write down your thoughts in your Intuitive Arts notebook about what the astrological sign and house placements of the Tarot cards for each heavenly body reveal to you about your health.

Intuition Rising: A Body, Mind, and Spirit Scan

In Chapter 1, we introduced you to the practice of using body scan and breath awareness to bring relaxation to different parts of your body. In this exercise, we use body scan, breath awareness, and the Tarot to help you create an intuition scan of your body, mind, and spirit.

Remember our energy word chart in Chapter 6? We are going to ask you to assign a different energy word to each part as you scan through your body. Then we ask you to assign a Tarot card to each part, much like you did in the previous exercise.

Okay, are you ready? Get in a comfortable place, somewhere where it is quiet with no distractions. Start by looking at the table showing which area of the body is ruled by which astrological sign. As you get to each one, visualize that part of your body in your mind's eye, tuning in to its energy. Visualize the ways it functions and the gifts it brings to you. Take in a deep breath or two. Now jot down an energy word. Go through your Tarot deck, reciting this energy word as a mantra. For instance, if you picked "expanding" for your brain, say this word again and again as you select a card from the deck. Place the card in front of you.

Work your way through each body part, taking the time to breathe deeply and relax your "thinking" mind.

Body Part	Astro Sign	Energy Word	My Tarot Card
Eyes	Aries ♈	_____	_____
Brain	Aries ♈	_____	_____
Throat, neck	Taurus ♉	_____	_____
Thyroid	Taurus ♉	_____	_____
Shoulders and arms	Gemini ♊	_____	_____

Body Part	Astro Sign	Energy Word	My Tarot Card
Spine, upper back	Leo ♌	_____	_____
Heart	Leo ♌	_____	_____
Stomach	Cancer ♋	_____	_____
Breasts	Cancer ♋	_____	_____
Intestines, colon	Virgo ♍	_____	_____
Lower back	Libra ♎	_____	_____
Kidneys	Libra ♎	_____	_____
Genitals	Scorpio ♏	_____	_____
Urinary tract	Scorpio ♏	_____	_____
Pelvis, hips, thighs	Sagittarius ♐	_____	_____
Liver	Sagittarius ♐	_____	_____
Skeleton, bones	Capricorn ♑	_____	_____
Calves, ankles	Aquarius ♒	_____	_____
Circulatory system	Aquarius ♒	_____	_____
Immune system	Pisces ♓	_____	_____
Hormone system	Pisces ♓	_____	_____
Feet	Pisces ♓	_____	_____

We're almost there! Let's do the mind-spirit scan, using the seven chakras we learned about in Chapter 6. We remind you of the colors because we think it will help you visualize chakra energy.

Chakras	Center	Color	Energy Word	My Tarot Card
1st (Root)	Base of spine	Red	_____	_____
2nd (Desire)	Genitals	Orange	_____	_____
3rd (Power)	Solar plexus	Yellow	_____	_____
4th (Love)	Heart	Green	_____	_____

Chakras	Center	Color	Energy Word	My Tarot Card
5th (Expression)	Throat	Blue	_____	_____
6th (Intuition)	Third eye	Indigo	_____	_____
7th (Spirit)	Crown	Violet	_____	_____

Now take a few minutes to put it all together, analyzing the potential alive in each Tarot card. Make a few notes here.

_____

_____

Suit Yourself: Tarot Power Portrait

With your Vital Signs Portrait and your intuition scan, you have a good strong foundation for creating a big-picture plan for your health. Here, we show you a way to do health maintenance. We will bring in what we have learned about the Elements and *yin/yang* to describe your daily health challenges and resources.

For this exercise, we use only the Minor Arcana. Divide the cards into the four suits. Wands represent your power around your health. Cups reveal the state of your emotions and how they influence your health. Swords show you whether your struggles with pain are in your past or lie ahead, while Pentacles reveal the resources you have at your disposal to create your best picture of health.

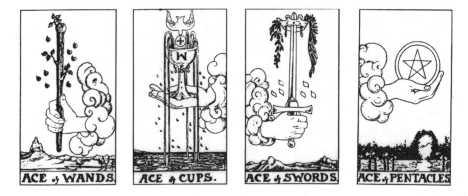

In the Minor Arcana, Wands represent your health power; Cups, your emotions; Swords, your pain and struggles; and Pentacles, your health resources.

If you'll remember from Chapters 2 and 3, each suit corresponds to *yin/yang* energy and the Elements. They also correspond to the energy of the chakras. Here's a quick review.

Tarot Deck

Suit	Health	Chakra	Energy	Element
Wands	Power	3rd (solar plexus) 1st (root)	*Yang*	Fire
Cups	Emotions	4th (heart) 2nd (desire)	*Yin*	Water
Swords	Pain	6th (third eye) 5th (throat)	*Yang*	Air
Pentacles	Resources	1st (root)	*Yin*	Earth

For the question to the suit of Wands, ask *"What is my power today around my health?"* For Cups, ask *"Where is the love and compassion in my life today in regard to my health?"* To Swords, ask *"What are my struggles today, and how should I respond to them?"* (Remember from Chapter 5, that pain and struggles can be the compass pointing to your soft spot, the place from which you forgive yourself and others.) To the Pentacles, ask *"Where are my resources for my health? Where should I turn?"*

For this exercise, shuffle each of the four decks and select a card from each, as in a Tarot reading. This reading is a handy tool to use for quick insight into how to approach your health and well-being each day. It can help you balance your *yin/yang* and your Elements. If, for instance, you don't have water in your three astrological power points (like Carolyn), you know already that you need to seek ways to cultivate water in your life, through the foods you eat, the exercises you choose, and the practices you use to soothe your soul. The card that comes up in your suit of Cups can point the way, and you'll also want to explore how (and whether) you are using *yin* effectively in your situation and to meditate on the fourth and second chakras.

Cups card: _____   Wands card: _____

Swords card: _____   Pentacles card: _____

Knowing where your health power and resources lie is like knowing what to pack for an African safari—only the adventure you seek is all the possibilities for your life once you have tapped into your optimum health. Now that we have everything packed in the suitcase, let's see what challenges await in the wild kingdom.

The Wild Kingdom: Challenges and Opportunities

As we have learned throughout this book, challenges take many forms in your astrological birth chart. We have learned about your Saturn ♄ return, your Pluto ♀ transit, the lessons of your North Node ☊, personal retrogrades, and the hidden challenges of your 12th house. In Chapter 4, we explored Astrology's aspects—the relationships between planets in your birth chart. As you may recall, squares □ and oppositions ☍ represent challenges and we focus on those here for this exercise.

Squares □ Considered to be challenging. Their tension often yields dramatic action in your life. Degree: 90°

Oppositions ☍ Like *yin* and *yang*, opposing planets show the need for balance between two competing energies. Degree: 180°

Where do squares □ and oppositions ☍ appear in your astrological birth chart? Identify these aspects by looking for their symbols in the triangular aspect grid, or in the center of your birth chart wheel. Do these challenging aspects involve your Sun ☉, Moon ☽, and ascendant, your astrological power points? Do they involve Jupiter ♃, the planet of expansion (sometimes literally, meaning weight gain!) or Saturn ♄, the planet of self-discipline? Do they involve Mars ♂ and the way you handle your anger? Look back to the beginning of this chapter for the reference table listing the heavenly bodies and their influence on your well-being. List a few of your square and oppositions here and make notes as to their meaning, either here or in your Intuitive Arts notebook. For example, ♂ □ ♃ could indicate that you are prone to explosive bursts of anger or unusually passionate responses that may surprise and confuse others—and even yourself! Your challenge is to use this energy for your health benefit, and not as a depleting force. Make a note of whether any of these challenging aspects involves 12th house planets; you can see this by looking at the aspect lines in the center of your birth chart wheel that show the aspects between the planets in their houses (in this case, the 12th house).

Your Squares □ and Oppositions ☍	Potential Meaning for Change and Rebalance
_____	_____
_____	_____
_____	_____

To create health opportunities, we can look at where the good-luck planet Jupiter ♃ appears in your astrological birth chart. We can peek inside the 10th house, the house of your ambitions, your highest aspirations, and your attainment. The 10th house is known as the house of success because it has goal-oriented Capricorn ♑ on its cusp and is ruled by serious, responsible Saturn ♄. This is where you get a chance to make it all happen—to be the healthiest you. Your 11th house is the house of hopes, wishes, and friends, the place where your allies can help you make your dreams come true. Conjunctions ☌ are two planets who are allies, combining their energy for your benefit. Conjunctions in your 10th or 11th houses should make you stand up and take note! We'll also be looking for the trines △ and sextiles ✶ in your astrological birth chart.

Conjunctions ☌ The strongest of the aspects.

Trines △ Considered the most favorable aspects. Their signs usually share the same element: Air, Fire, Water, Earth. Degree: 120°

Sextiles ✶ Considered harmonious. These bring about opportunities and attract possibilities. Degree: 60°

Where do conjunctions ☌, trines △, and sextiles ✶ appear? Do these opportunistic aspects involve your Sun ☉, Moon ☽, and ascendant, your astrological power points? And of course Jupiter ♃ and Saturn ♄? Do they involve Venus ♀ and Neptune ♆, the planets of compassion and forgiveness? Look back again, if you need to, for the reference table listing the heavenly bodies and their influence on your well-being. List a few of your conjunctions, trines, and sextiles here and make notes as to their meaning, either here or in your Intuitive Arts notebook. Make a particular note if any of these beneficial aspects appear in your 10th or 11th houses.

Your Conjunctions ☌, Trines △, and Sextiles ✶	Potential Meaning for Health Opportunities
_____	_____
_____	_____
_____	_____

Briefly, let's return to the birth chart of poet Maya Angelou, whom we first encountered in Chapter 1.

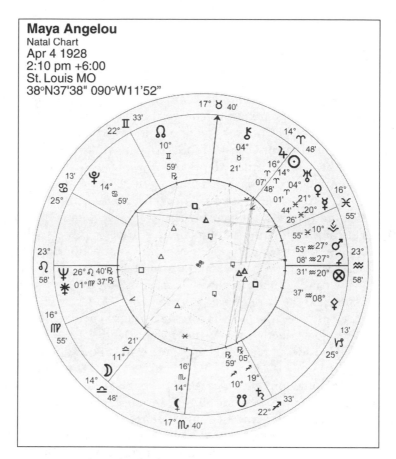

Maya Angelou's birth chart.

In Maya's Saturn ♄ squares □, to Mercury ☿ and to Venus ♀, we find she would face grave challenges in personal relationships and the need to express those struggles. Her parents divorced when she was two, and she was sexually assaulted at age eight, remaining silent for four years. But because she has a Mercury conjunct Venus ☿ ☌ ♀, Maya possessed the ability to convey her personal heartaches to others in a way that touched them. That influence equipped her to be reflective about her challenges and urged her to express them through creative outlets, which are dominant in her birth chart. Maya's chart has many

Mercury and Venus influences, as well as the intuitive, artistic sign of Pisces ♓.

Pluto ♀ is square □ with her Aries ♈ Sun ☉, which presents challenges to her in society or family conditioning. This square may have caused Maya frustration as a young girl until she went inward and transformed herself, which may explain the role her four years of silence played in shaping the poet we know now. This influence may also have forced her into the public arena, even if she shunned the spotlight. Born Marguerite Johnson, she first "became" Maya Angelou when she performed at the Purple Onion nightclub in San Francisco in 1953. Her Pluto ♀ square □ to her natal Moon ☽ in Libra ♎ and natal Sun ☉ in Aries ♈ points to her need to gain freedom from past losses and transform herself completely.

Among Maya's favorable aspects are Saturn trine Sun ♄ △ ☉, Saturn trine Jupiter ♄ △ ♃, and Saturn trine Neptune ♄ △ ♆. These show she would be able to transform a negative aspect into positive application of personal awareness and want to share that self-awareness with others. Saturn trine Sun is a natural-born teacher, while Saturn trine Neptune is a natural-born artist with a gift for self-expression and spiritual insight into the human desire to evolve beyond limitations.

Emerging Patterns: A Tarot Analysis

An analysis of all of the Tarot readings you have done so far for this book can help you see what patterns are emerging. If you are like Carolyn, you may get so many "a-ha moments" from a Tarot reading that you aren't sure where to begin. Doing a card analysis periodically using your Intuitive Arts notebook can help you see common themes that come up. If you see a particular message again and again, that's the one to focus on first. After all, we don't expect you to drop all salt and sugar from your diet, eat more steamed vegetables, start a weight-training program, join a tai chi class, meditate daily, and heal your relationship with your mother all at once!

A Tarot card analysis looks at these factors:

- **Your most common card.** This card will have special meaning in your life. Pay special attention to the archetypes to master the qualities they represent. This is like hitting the mother lode to your personal power.
- **Dominant suit.** The suit from the Minor Arcana that shows up most often.

- **Dominant Element—Fire, Water, Air, or Earth.** Each suit of the Minor Arcana matches up with an Element. This is the Element that shows up most often.
- **Astrological influences.** This looks at the astrological influences reflected in the Major Arcana cards that have come up in your series of readings. For how the Major Arcana reflect astrological influences, look back to Chapter 3.
- **Numerological influences.** Look through the Minor Arcana in your readings to find the most frequently recurring numbers.

When Carolyn did a Tarot card analysis, she found it very revealing.

Most common Tarot card: 3 of Cups. The 3 of Cups points immediately to Carolyn's three sisters, who provide the core of her identity and her emotional support. They are her best advocates. The way the three women are dancing, in grace, harmony, and celebration, is the way she feels when she is with her sisters. This image has long been a power image for Carolyn. She has a portrait of the Three Graces from Sandro Botticelli's painting *Primavera* in her house.

Dominant suit: Cups. This indicates Carolyn listens with her heart; she has tapped into a source of compassion within.

Dominant Element: Water. This calls Carolyn to listen with more sensitivity to her own emotional needs, to do more feeling than thinking.

Astrological influences. Sign: Taurus ♉. Taurus, the sign of security, directs Carolyn to put down deep roots and build a strong foundation for her life. (She had just emerged from a divorce.) It indicates that Carolyn, a Sagittarian ♐ who thrives on adventure and is often restless for change and exploration, needs to focus on security. Knowing that she has a safety net in place will be vital to a healthy body, mind, and spirit.

Planet: The Sun ☉. Because the Sun is the center of the solar system and the core of our identity, this indicates that Carolyn is being called to clarify her deepest understanding of her personal purpose.

Numerological influences: 3. The 3 in Carolyn's analysis indicates the need for creative self-expression. The message to Carolyn is to free herself from rules and expectations from childhood that might be restricting her expression.

A Year of Health: Tarot's Horoscope Spread

Now, roll up your sleeves and let's get to work on a plan for your health for the next 12 months. Tarot's Horoscope Spread provides you with a comprehensive portrait of your health in body, mind, and spirit and signal guideposts for your journey. Each of the cards in the Horoscope Spread corresponds with the 12 houses on the astrological wheel. As you choose a card for each house, place it in the appropriate position.

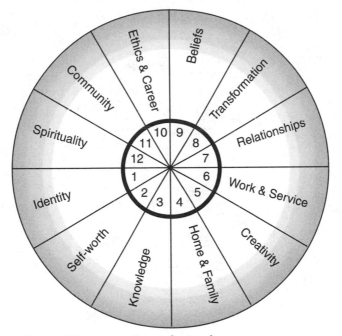

Tarot's Horoscope Spread reveals your comprehensive wellness plan for your health in the coming 12 months.

For this Tarot reading, ask for clear instruction in the steps ahead to take positive action for your health. The cards may tell you that you need to set up some best practices in your life for health—changing your diet or exercising more. Or your reading may reveal that something in your emotional or spiritual life needs to be addressed before you can move forward. Use the following table for clues as to the interpretations of each of the 12 cards you chose.

House	Arena of Life	Planetary Ruler	Chakra	How It Relates to Your Health
1st	Self, ego	Aries ♈	1 (root), 3 (power)	Body / Your constitution
2nd	Life values, possessions, sensuality	Taurus ♉	2 (desire)	Body / Your health blessings / Resources that support your health
3rd	Self-expression, communication, memory, logic	Gemini ♊	3 (power), 5 (expression)	Mind / Healthy communication / Being understood, ability to learn, making decisions
4th	Home, family of origin, roots	Cancer ♋	1 (root), 4 (heart)	Mind / Your relationships, your emotional wounds
5th	Creativity, sexuality, risk-taking, children	Leo ♌	6 (intuition), 7 (spirituality)	Spirit / Your spiritual legacy
6th	Service	Virgo ♍	2 (desire), 4 (heart)	Spirit / Your mission in life / How you balance work and health
7th	Marriage, partnership	Libra ♎	2 (desire), 4 (heart)	Mind, spirit / Your ability to set aside selfish needs for the good of another; your ability to sustain shared goals and visions with another
8th	Resources, money, life force	Scorpio ♏	2 (desire), 6 (third eye)	Mind, spirit / Your passion; your shadows; your temptations; your ability to transform yourself
9th	Higher knowledge, spirituality	Sagittarius ♐	7 (spirituality)	Spirit / Your spiritual quest
10th	Your reputation, your career	Capricorn ♑	5 (expression), 7 (spirituality)	Body / Your highest potential
11th	Hopes and dreams, friends and alliances	Aquarius ♒	4 (heart), 6 (third eye)	Mind / Your vision
12th	Subconscious	Pisces ♓	6 (third eye), 7 (spirituality)	Spirit / Your instincts and intuition

To deepen your understanding of your Horoscope Spread, return to the Tarot touchstones you did in Chapter 4, which helped you identify the best practices for your health, self-esteem, and spirit. There, we walked you through questions about shoring up the areas of your life that support your health. Here's a quick review:

Tarot Touchstones

1 Nurturing positive relationships

2 Nurturing positive careers

3 Nurturing personal growth

4 Nurturing home

5 Changing your energy

6 Radiating positive energy

Draw upon the Tarot touchstones as you take notes on your horoscope reading. For instance, if a card that turns up for one of the houses—say your 4th house of emotional wounds or your 7th house of partnership—feels perplexing, exciting, or disturbing to you, take it as a sign to go deeper. Do this by drawing a few more Tarot cards with more focused, specific questions. Examples might be, "Is this conflict with my soulmate or my family of origin?" or "How can I build around me a family of the heart?" Then, deeper: "How is this conflict or this lack diminishing my health?" Deeper still: "What would help me take the first step in changing this?" This can aid you in fleshing out an action plan.

Know also that Tarot's Horoscope Spread can be a month-by-month guide, giving you practical insight about when to begin focusing on that area of your health. That is, you may find that the time to take action on addressing the emotional wounds in your 4th house is indeed the 4th month of your plan.

House	Area of Influence	Possible Action Plan
1st	Your constitution	Your diet, your exercise plan
2nd	Your health blessings	Make a list of your body's strengths
3rd	Your communication style; the way you talk, the way you listen	Work on listening skills; work on expression skills
4th	Your emotional wounds	Look up a long-lost friend; find new ways of talking to a

House	Area of Influence	Possible Action Plan
		parent or sibling who hurt you; explore your childhood
5th	Your courage, your children; your creativity	Take a chance; try a new vitamin regimen or exercise plan; spend more time with your children; take a water color or pottery class
6th	Your mission in life	Volunteer for a cause; give one Saturday a month; start a support group; raise money for a charity
7th	Your sharing style	Working on your marriage; building a support network; forging a partnership
8th	Your temptations, your capacity for change	Identify weaknesses and work to conquer one of them; collect success stories of people who changed their health dramatically
9th	Your quest for higher knowledge	Do research on homeopathy, aromatherapy, vitamins, nutrition
10th	Your career, your highest potential	Change career; ask for a raise; start a business that supports your highest values; put your ideas out there in the form of a book or nonprofit cause
11th	Your vision, and your vision-keepers	Write out your vision; make a list of your vision-keepers
12th	Your instincts, your intuition your hidden challenges	Tune in to your instincts; learn to act on them

For fun, Arlene and Carolyn did Horoscope Spreads, mapping out a 12-month game plan for our health. It's sort of like New Year's resolutions (in print!), so we'll both be checking back in to see how we did.

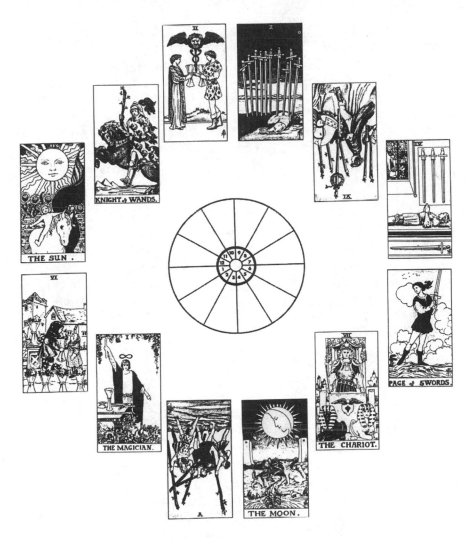

Arlene's Horoscope Reading.

House	Area of Influence	Arlene's Tarot Card	Arlene's Action Plan
1st	Your constitution	6 of Cups	**Optimism** Maintain harmony with my inner child; maintain positive outlook

House	Area of Influence	Arlene's Tarot Card	Arlene's Action Plan
2nd	Your health blessings	The Magician	**Heal thyself** Know and appreciate my innate healing power; be grateful for my ability to bounce back quickly
3rd	Your communication style; the way you talk, the way you listen	5 of Wands R	**Harmony/peace** Focus on communicating through conflict with positive attitude
4th	Your emotional wounds	The Moon	**Emotional attunement** Reflect on the past, heal any emotional ties
5th	Your courage, your children, creativity	The Chariot	**Thrive** Know that I have good stamina, inner strength; as I face difficulties, visualize victory
6th	Your mission in life	Page of Swords	**Guard what I know** Be cautious about health and always seek deeper meanings to health issues
7th	Your sharing style	4 of Swords	**Meditate** Relax, take a break after emerging from difficult times; take time to reflect
8th	Your temptations, your capacity for change	6 of Wands R	**Lack of discipline** I need to be aware that I can stay stuck in old habits
9th	Your quest for higher knowledge	10 of Swords	**End old patterns** Find out all I can about health and wellness; complete my knowledge
10th	Your career, your highest potential	2 of Cups	**Contentment** Count my blessings in career and the partners I have there

House	Area of Influence	Arlene's Tarot Card	Arlene's Action Plan
11th	Your vision, and your vision-keepers	Knight of Wands	**Enthusiasm** Advance toward your new goals
12th	Your instincts, your intuition, own hidden challenges	The Sun	**Vitality** Pay attention to my light; develop and use positive affirmations

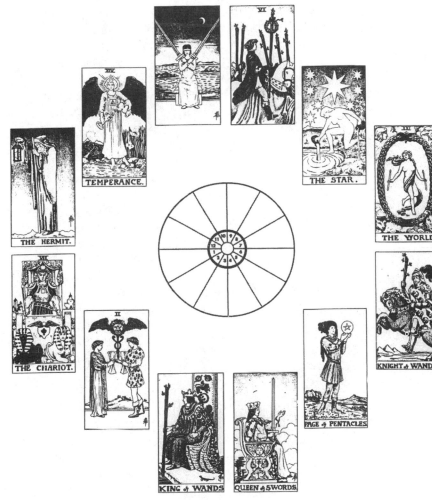

Carolyn's Horoscope Reading.

House	Area of Influence	Carolyn's Tarot Card	Carolyn's Action Plan
1st	Your constitution	The Chariot	**Thrive** Gain stamina, strength, victory in establishing good health routine, be more diligent about taking vitamins, osteo-porosis prevention measures
2nd	Your health blessings	2 of Cups	**Count my blessings** Treasure friendships, alliances, support network; be good to them; treasure good health with best prac-tices of good nights' sleep, healthy diet; treat myself with loving kindness
3rd	Your communi-cation style; the way you talk, the way you listen	King of Wands	**Speak truth and clarity** Rely on gift of clear speaking, healthy communication, good listening; encourage growth in others through leadership
4th	Your emotional wounds	Queen of Swords	**The truth will set you free** Bear sorrows well, heal relationships with penetrating words of truth, keen observa-tions, sympathetic listening, solid logic
5th	Your courage, your children, creativity	Page of Pentacles	**Slow down** Spend more time with my children, learn about slowing down and taking care of myself through them

House	Area of Influence	Carolyn's Tarot Card	Carolyn's Action Plan
6th	Your mission in life	Knight of Wands	**Woman with a mission** Know I have the power to manifest my dreams, my true purpose
7th	Your sharing style	The World	**Attainment** Find clarity about the role of partnership in my life; know I will triumph in my quest; liberate myself from chains of past mistakes
8th	Your temptations, your capacity for change	The Star	**Open heart chakra** Cultivate power of intent; give and receive love
9th	Your quest for higher knowledge	6 of Wands	**Lessons learned well** Battle is won; victory is mine; success is around the corner
10th	Your career, your highest potential	2 of Swords	**Breakthrough time** Overcome indecision about career direction
11th	Your vision, and your vision-keepers	Temperance	**Discipline** Have patience for unfolding of my dreams; have more self-discipline; cultivate vision-keepers
12th	Your instincts, your intuition, own hidden challenges	The Hermit	**Intuition is my friend** Take time out to listen to my inner voice

Now it's your turn.

House	Area of Influence	Your Tarot Card	Your Action Plan
1st	_____	_____	_____
2nd	_____	_____	_____
3rd	_____	_____	_____
4th	_____	_____	_____
5th	_____	_____	_____
6th	_____	_____	_____
7th	_____	_____	_____
8th	_____	_____	_____
9th	_____	_____	_____
10th	_____	_____	_____
11th	_____	_____	_____
12th	_____	_____	_____

Entering the Bliss Center of Health

In Tibetan Buddhism, the mandala is an imaginary palace that you contemplate during meditation practice. Each object in the palace has significance, representing some guiding principle. Each mandala is different, with different lessons to learn. Mandala is Sanskrit for *circle, community,* and *connection*—and a mandala signifies the wholeness of eternity. The pupil must cross the threshold of each palace circle, having learned its lesson, before progressing to the center.

In a mandala inspired by Jytte Hansen of Denmark (www.jyh.dk/indengl.htm#Mandala), the outermost circle is the **fire of wisdom,** and it consists of purifying fire. This is the innocent, exploring energy of Tarot's Fool transformed into wisdom attained in the World. The next circle is called the *vajra* circle, or **diamond circle,** which expresses strength and fearlessness. This is the stage of spiritual development where you gather your fortitude—becoming as hard and as beautiful as a polished diamond. The third circle is composed of the **tombs,** symbolizing the eight stages of consciousness: seeing, hearing, tasting, smelling, body, thinking, "I," and core consciousness. Finally, there is the **lotus circle**, the ultimate destination, in which the heart and spirit express an open state of devotion and enter into eternal enlightenment.

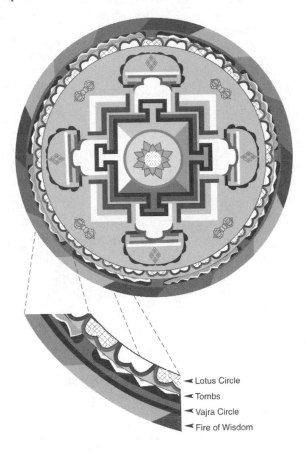

The mandala is a path to bliss.

For this exercise, we use the Buddhist mandala to guide you to spiritual health, manifest your highest intentions, transcend your inner demons, and tap into your most heartfelt dreams. We help you see your choices for the infinite and manifest them, setting you firmly on the path to a beautiful eternity.

As you contemplate the mandala, visualize yourself floating through each of the circles, entering the rooms of a beautiful palace that a benevolent and loving force has provided for you. As you move toward the mandala's center, meditate upon the message of each circle:

- ☯ **Fire of Wisdom:** exploring innocence transformed into wisdom
- ☯ **Diamond:** fortitude, strength, fearlessness
- ☯ **Tombs:** see, hear, taste, smell, the physical body, the thinking mind, "I," your core consciousness
- ☯ **Lotus:** enlightenment, bliss.

As you approach the mandala's center through each of its circles, prompt your intuitive heart with the following visualizations:

- ☯ What do you want to manifest in your life? Visualize yourself as the healthiest person you can be. What do you look like? How do you move? How do you talk to others? How do you listen?
- ☯ What are you actively trying to achieve with your health? These are your specific goals and the actions you take to work on them. See yourself accomplishing your goals.
- ☯ What beliefs hinder you? What negative people diminish you? What positive people lift you up and nurture your soul?
- ☯ What resources do you have in you to accomplish your goals? What particular qualities do you bring that are your unique gifts? This moves you toward the diamond circle, the place where you become hard and beautiful.
- ☯ What sorrows are holding you back? What do you need to grieve? This is the walk through the tombs in the mandala. Visualize what has passed from you—people you have loved, pursuits you have loved but no longer make you thrive.
- ☯ How do you view yourself now, in this present moment? How do you *want* to view yourself?
- ☯ What is your true purpose?

Now, you are there at the center, standing at the vital bliss point of optimal mind, body, and spirit health. We hope that, using the Intuitive Arts as your guide, you may return to this sacred place of well-being again and again.

appendix A

Vital Stars

The Wheel of the Zodiac
By the signs
By the planets
Planetary rulers
House keywords
Asteroids and Planetoids
Aspects
Vital signs
Ordering birth charts and synastry grids online

We've pulled together all of the Astrology basics in one quick-reference guide. Use it to help you navigate Astrology's signs, planets, and houses as you look into your astrological birth chart for your picture of health and well-being.

The Wheel of the Zodiac

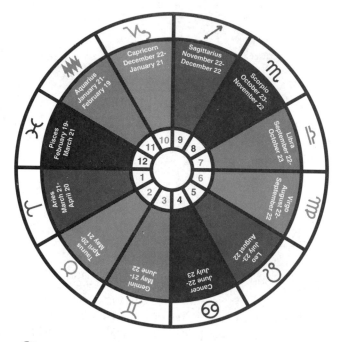

By the Signs

Here's a quick, handy reference to the astrological signs.

Aries, the Ram ♈   March 21 to April 20

Element	Fire
Quality	Cardinal
Energy	*Yang*
Rulers	Mars and Pluto
Anatomy	Brain, eyes, face
Keywords	Pioneering, initiating, beginnings

Taurus, the Bull ♉   April 20 to May 21

Element	Earth
Quality	Fixed
Energy	*Yin*
Ruler	Venus
Anatomy	Neck, throat, thyroid
Keywords	Ownership, dependability, sensuality

Gemini, the Twins ♊ May 21 to June 22

Element	Air
Quality	Mutable
Energy	*Yang*
Ruler	Mercury
Anatomy	Hands, arms, shoulders, lungs
Keywords	Mentality, communication, versatility

Cancer, the Crab ♋ June 22 to July 23

Element	Water
Quality	Cardinal
Energy	*Yin*
Ruler	Moon
Anatomy	Stomach, breasts
Keywords	Feeling, sensitivity, nurturing

Leo, the Lion ♌ July 23 to August 22

Element	Fire
Quality	Fixed
Energy	*Yang*
Ruler	Sun
Anatomy	Back, spine, heart
Keywords	Willpower, creativity, expressing the heart

Virgo, the Virgin ♍ August 22 to September 22

Element	Earth
Quality	Mutable
Energy	*Yin*
Ruler	Mercury
Anatomy	Intestines and colon
Keywords	Service, self-improvement, sacred patterns

Libra, the Scales ♎ September 22 to October 23

Element	Air
Quality	Cardinal
Energy	*Yang*
Ruler	Venus
Anatomy	Kidneys, lower back, adrenal glands
Keywords	Balance, harmony, justice

Scorpio, the Scorpion ♏

	October 23 to November 22
Element	Water
Quality	Fixed
Energy	*Yin*
Rulers	Pluto and Mars
Anatomy	Genitals, urinary and reproductive systems
Keywords	Desire, transformation, power

Sagittarius, the Archer ♐

	November 22 to December 22
Element	Fire
Quality	Mutable
Energy	*Yang*
Ruler	Jupiter
Anatomy	Liver, hips, thighs
Keywords	Discovery, truth-seeking, enthusiasm

Capricorn, the Goat ♑

	December 22 to January 21
Element	Earth
Quality	Cardinal
Energy	*Yin*
Ruler	Saturn
Anatomy	Bones, joints, knees, teeth
Keywords	Achievement, structure, responsibility

Aquarius, the Water Bearer ♒

	January 21 to February 19
Element	Air
Quality	Fixed
Energy	*Yang*
Rulers	Uranus and Saturn
Anatomy	Ankles, circulation
Keywords	Humanitarian, unique, innovative

Pisces, the Fishes ♓

	February 19 to March 21
Element	Water
Quality	Mutable
Energy	*Yin*

Pisces, the Fishes ♓	February 19 to March 21
Rulers	Neptune and Jupiter
Anatomy	Feet, immune system, hormonal system
Keywords	Compassion, universality, inclusiveness

By the Planets

Here's a quick, handy reference to the energy of each planet.

Planet	Symbol	Energies	Action Keyword
Sun	☉	Self, essence, life spirit, creativity, willpower	Explores
Moon	☽	Emotions, instincts, unconscious, past memories	Senses
Mercury	☿	Mental activities, communication, intelligence	Communicates
Venus	♀	Love, art, beauty, social graces, harmony, money, resources, possessions	Enjoys
Mars	♂	Physical energy, boldness, warrior ways, action, desires anger, courage, ego	Acts
Jupiter	♃	Luck, abundance, wisdom, higher education, philosophy or beliefs, exploration, growth	Benefits
Saturn	♄	Responsibilities, self-discipline, perseverance, limitations, structures	Works
Uranus	♅	Sudden or unexpected change, originality, liberation, radical thinking, authenticity	Innovates
Neptune	♆	Idealism, subconscious, spirituality, intuition, clairvoyance	Dreams
Pluto	♇	Power, regeneration, destruction, rebirth, transformation	Transforms

Signs in Houses

House	Astro Sign
1st	Aries ♈
2nd	Taurus ♉
3rd	Gemini ♊
4th	Cancer ♋
5th	Leo ♌
6th	Virgo ♍
7th	Libra ♎
8th	Scorpio ♏
9th	Sagittarius ♐
10th	Capricorn ♑
11th	Aquarius ♒
12th	Pisces ♓

Planetary Rulers

Planet	Signs Ruled
Sun ☉	Leo ♌
Moon ☽	Cancer ♋
Mercury ☿	Gemini ♊, Virgo ♍
Venus ♀	Taurus ♉, Libra ♎
Mars ♂	Aries ♈, co-ruler of Scorpio ♏
Jupiter ♃	Sagittarius ♐, co-ruler of Pisces ♓
Saturn ♄	Capricorn ♑, co-ruler of Aquarius ♒
Uranus ♅	Aquarius ♒
Neptune ♆	Pisces ♓
Pluto ♇	Scorpio ♏, co-ruler of Aries ♈

House Key Terms

House	Key Term
1st	Identity
2nd	Self-worth
3rd	Knowledge
4th	Home and family
5th	Creativity
6th	Work and service
7th	Relationships

House	Key Term
8th	Transformation
9th	Beliefs
10th	Ethics and career
11th	Community
12th	Spirituality

Natural Planets and Natural Signs in Their Houses

Here are the natural planets and natural signs in their astrological houses.

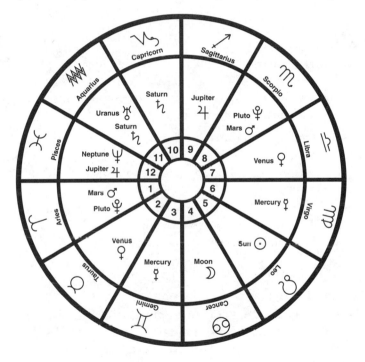

Asteroids and Planetoids

In Chapter 8, we discussed in detail the asteroid Ceres ⚳ and planetoid Chiron ⚷, which influence your spiritual health. Here's a look at all of the asteroids, plus Chiron, and what they represent.

Asteroid	Realm	Areas of Influence
Ceres ⚳	Motherhood	Natural cycles, fertility, crops, relationships between parents and children
Juno ⚵	Marriage	Partnerships, contracts and agreements, social obligations
Pallas Athene ⚴	Wisdom	Intelligence, knowledge, understanding, equality
Vesta ⚶	Power	Sexuality, devotion, health, service to others
Planetoid		
Chiron ⚷	Healing	Transformation, personal growth

Aspects

Aspects are the geometric relationships between any two planets in your own chart, as well as in relation to another chart, whether for another person, a moment in time, or your own progressed chart. The main aspects to consider are as follows:

- **Conjunction** ☌ The strongest aspects. In a conjunction, the planets are placed at the same point on a chart or charts. Conjunctions are considered a focal point, with the interaction of the two planets emphasized.
- **Sextile** ✶ In a sextile, the planets are 60° apart. The signs in a sextile share the same energy (*yin* or *yang*), so this is considered to be a favorable aspect.
- **Square** □ In a square, the planets are 90° apart. While squares are considered to be chart challenges, they often provide the impetus for change and improvement.
- **Trine** △ In a trine, the planets are 120° apart. This most favorable of the aspects means the planets share both element and energy. Trines indicate positive connections, often made so easily you might not even notice.
- **Opposition** ☍ In an opposition, the planets are 180° apart. There's little in common with an opposition, but, like squares, their difficult energy can spur us on to meet challenges.
- **Quincunx** ⚻ In a quincunx, the planets are 150° apart. Quincunxes are interesting—nothing is shared between the two signs, so some adjustment is usually required in order for them to interact.

Astrological Extras

The astrological charts and grids you see as examples throughout this book contain two symbols we don't include in our discussions but that might interest you in your further explorations of Astrology. These are the Part of Fortune ⊗ and the minor asteroid Lilith ⚸. The Part of Fortune, sometimes called the Lot of Fortune, derives from ancient Astrology and represents the intersection in the Zodiac where your Sun ☉, Moon ☽, and ascendant converge. The Part of Fortune in its basic symbolism is a "point of karmic reward" in your birth chart. The ancients believed the Part of Fortune is what you would receive as a cosmic gift as you grew in this lifetime. Lilith, also called the Dark Moon, represents primal and emotional connections to your shadow side, and "liberation from conformity" in present-day interpretations.

Vital Signs

Health and vitality abound in your astrological birth chart. Here's a quick guide to key power points in your chart.

1. In Chapter 1, we showed you where to look for your Sun ☉ sign. Each Sun ☉ sign rules a part of your body, and each has its own vulnerabilities.

2. In Chapter 2, you learned about your *yin/yang* equation: which signs have a *yin* quality and which have a *yang* quality. We introduced the Moon ☽ sign, which rules your emotions and how you sense the world. Because the Moon travels through a new constellation every 2½ days, it can influence the energy of a day.

3. In Chapter 3, we introduced you to your Elemental Health Signature. We looked at your astrological power points, adding in your ascendant with your Sun ☉ and Moon ☽ signs. We looked at how many power points you have in Fire, Earth, Air, and Water signs.

4. In Chapter 4, you learned how to look to the houses of the strongest health influences—the 1st, 4th, 6th, 7th, 10th and 12th—to get clues about your self-esteem and how it affects your health. We also counted astrological aspects to tally up planetary opportunities and challenges.

5. In Chapter 5, we introduced Venus ♀ and Neptune ♆, the two "soft spots" in your chart that reveal your forgiveness style. We also explored Astrology's synastry of health relationships.

6. In Chapter 6, we explored how Mars ♂ affects the way you deal with anger.

7. Also in Chapter 6, we walked you through how to cultivate a healthy sense of optimism by understanding how Jupiter ♃ influences you.

8. Also in Chapter 6, we showed you how personal retrogrades ℞ change the way the energy of a planet is expressed. Retrogrades are indicated in your aspect grid.

9. In Chapter 7, we showed you how to use an ephemeris to chart your year ahead so that you can work through the phases of grieving.

10. Also in Chapter 7, we showed you how to reveal the meaning of a Saturn ♄ return and a Pluto ♀ transit.

11. In Chapter 8, we explained the hidden challenges that lie in your 12th house and have implications for your soul in this life and beyond.

12. Also in Chapter 8, we elaborated on the role of the rising sign in pointing the way to your life lessons—the person you are becoming.

13. Also in Chapter 8, we explained the lessons of the North Node ☊ and South Node ☋, and looked at the karmic resonances in a progressed astrological chart.

14. Also in Chapter 8, we introduced you to the asteroids and Chiron ⚷, and showed you how they can guide you in healing your wounds and leaving a spiritual legacy.

15. In Chapter 9, we showed you how to explore beneficial and challenging planetary aspects for health in your astrological birth chart.

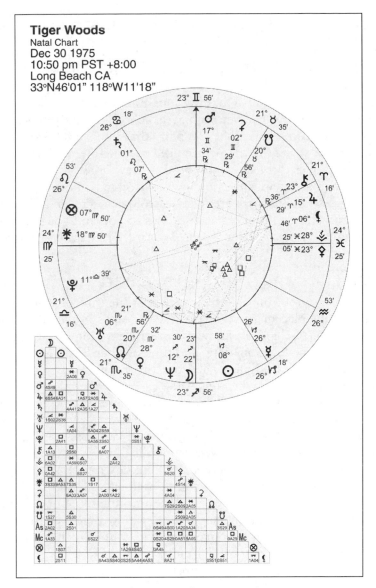

Tiger Woods's birth chart and aspect grid.

Ordering Birth Charts and Synastry Grids Online

Several websites will do birth charts for you. To get a birth chart you can use with this book, be sure to specify that you want Geocentric, Tropical Zodiac, Placidus House system, and True Node. Check out Arlene's site at www.mellinetti.com. Also check out Astrolabe, Inc., at www.alabe.com—this is the company that publishes Solar Fire, the computer software program Arlene used to generate the birth charts we used as examples throughout this book. A few other good Astrology websites include www.astro.com, www.astrodatabank.com, and www.stariq.com. But there are many astrological sites on the Internet; explore and choose the site that resonates to you and your investigation of Astrology, the heavens, and your *healthful* place in the universe.

Birth Time and Your Birth Chart

The position of the Sun ☉ in the heavens at the time of your birth determines the placement of the planets and signs in the houses of your astrological birth chart. To know the precise position of the Sun, you need to know the location, date, and time of your birth. Many people don't know their birth times. There are various methods astrologers can use to cast birth charts when this is the case.

For the birth charts with unknown birth times that we used in this book, Arlene used the method called "noon chart." A noon chart uses noon as your time of birth, placing your Sun ☉ at the apex of the horoscope wheel—on your midheaven. Symbolically, this puts your soul at its highest potential in this lifetime, looking down with an eagle's-eye view, so to speak, on the planets and how they "fall" into place in the astrological houses to represent your life. Although there are some imprecisions with this or any method of casting a birth chart without a precise time of birth (for example, the ascendant sign changes every two hours), Arlene finds the noon chart allows the most accurate interpretations for the broadest range of people.

appendix B

Vital Cards

The beauty of each Tarot card is that no card's meaning is absolute. Each is open to personal interpretation, and that means your Psychic Intuition is valuable as you study each card's individual image and contemplate the archetypes and stories depicted there. In this appendix, we give your intuition a boost by providing the traditional meanings of the cards—along with special meanings for body, mind, and spirit health. The images you see here are from the Universal Waite Tarot Deck, published by U.S. Games Systems, Inc. Start with this deck, or choose any of the many other Tarot decks available. You may want to explore the imagery of several decks as you learn and grow through the Tarot.

Tarot's Major Arcana

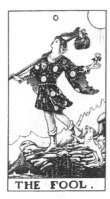

The Fool
A brand new start on health
Endless possibilities, optimism
Naivete and innocence
Open to a new health regimen

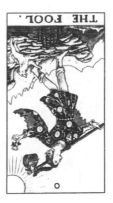

The Fool R
Uncertainty
A wrong direction
Ignoring health
Look before you leap!

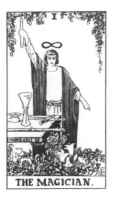

The Magician
The power to
manifest desire
Ask and ye shall
receive
A creative or
inventive person

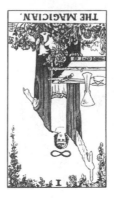

The Magician R
Possibility of
manipulation
Lack of follow-
through
A user or abuser

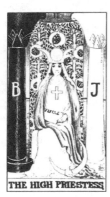

The High Priestess
Intuition and inner
knowing
Yin and yang;
emotions + logic
Your third eye

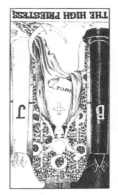

The High Priestess R
Dream or illusion
A hidden agenda
Lack of insight

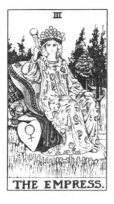

The Empress
A happy home
Harmony and
health
An environment
for growth and
prosperity

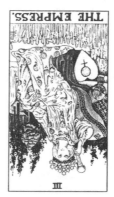

The Empress R
Disagreements
at home
Too much focus
on physical
appearance
Domination
rather than
dominion

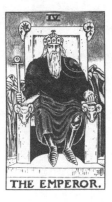

*The Emperor
Father figure
Past experience
can guide the
present
Self-discipline*

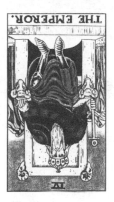

*The Emperor R
Insecurity
Stubbornness
Self-centeredness*

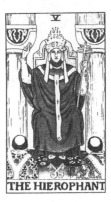

*The Hierophant
Adherence to tra-
ditional medicine
Staying between
the lines
A solid spiritual
foundation*

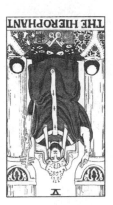

*The Hierophant R
Open to alternative
medicine
A risk-taker
A relationship with
freedom*

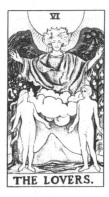

*The Lovers
A new alliance
Good start for
a new health
advocate
Peaceful coexis-
tence*

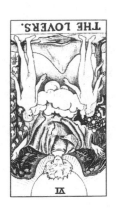

*The Lovers R
Separation or
division
Obstacles to desires
Need for better
emotional commu-
nication*

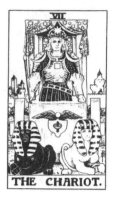

The Chariot
Ability to meet
challenges
Focus and deter-
mination to
achieve a goal
Positive outcome
after difficult
time
Healing and recu-
perating well

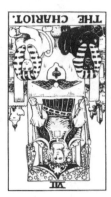

The Chariot R
Confusion
Someone else in
control
A battle not
worth fighting?
Need to monitor
health or recovery

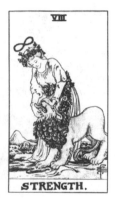

Strength
The inner strength
of unconditional
support
Love without fear
The power of
gentle persuasion
Strong constitu-
tion

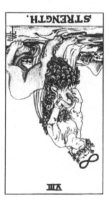

Strength R
A power struggle
Intense emotions
that can lead to
upset
Uncontrolled
passions
Lack of discipline

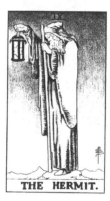

The Hermit
Introspection and
solitude
A desire for truth
Trust own inner
voice for guid-
ance

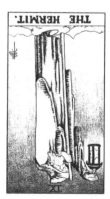

The Hermit R
Inability to see
clearly
Wishing instead
of acting
Not paying atten-
tion to medical
wisdom

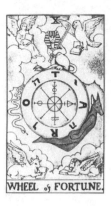

The Wheel of Fortune
Destiny comes calling!
Lucky in health
True health and good fortune come around

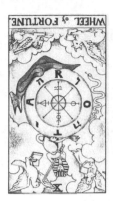

The Wheel of Fortune R
What goes up must come down
Good fortune in health slips away
Need to slow down and relax

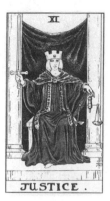

Justice
Fairness and a desire for balance
A legal agreement or alliance
Universal laws will prevail

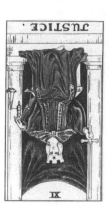

Justice R
Unwise counsel
Conditions that are out of balance
Too much subjectivity

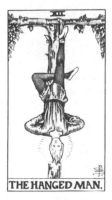

The Hanged Man
Relinquish old health habits
Need to reflect on the past, forgive
A lack of motion; feeling stuck

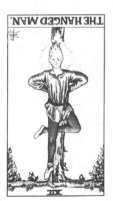

The Hanged Man R
Resistance to giving up old health habits
Holding on to the past
Fear of change

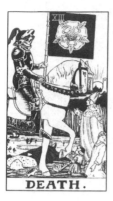

*Death
Renewal and
transformation
A catalyst for
change
A new dawn*

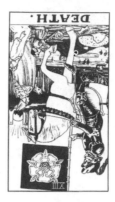

*Death R
Past blockages
impede progress
Stagnation and
stalemate
Arguments; too
tired to continue*

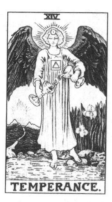

*Temperance
Balance between
emotion and
desire
Giving and taking
in equal measure
Moderation,
patience and
perseverance*

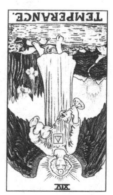

*Temperance R
Impatience
Inability to listen
to allies
Pushiness instead
of patience*

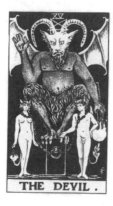

*The Devil
Obsessions,
weaknesses
Addictive
behaviors
Wrong applica-
tion of force,
aggression*

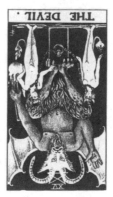

*The Devil R
Freedom from
fears or addiction
Ability to unlock
own chains
A burden lifted*

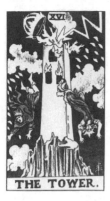

The Tower
Surprise!
Collapse of a
faulty foundation
Catharsis before
a new start

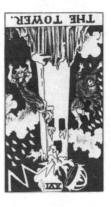

The Tower R
Surprising nuance
to a situation
Pay attention to
intuitive nudges
Renewed faith after
difficult life change

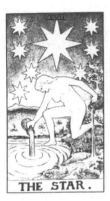

The Star
A faith in your
vitality
Giving and tak-
ing in balance
Abundance,
return of hope

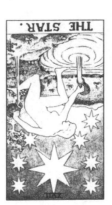

The Star R
Insecurity, giving
too much
Loss of hope, not
always warranted
Need to heal

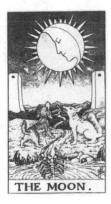

The Moon
Emotions at full
force
A reminder to
trust your psychic
intuition
Is someone hid-
ing something?

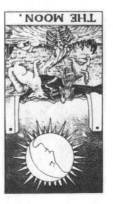

The Moon R
Understanding
after initial con-
fusion
Clarity of light
after darkness
Relief after worry

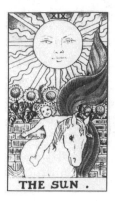

The Sun
Personal content-
ment, success
Sunny outlook
for health, possi-
ble pregnancy
Good self-esteem,
good self-
discipline

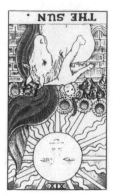

The Sun R
Diminished
vitality
Insecure or frag-
ile health
Cloudy forecast,
need counsel

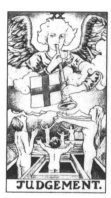

Judgement
A new under-
standing of past
lessons
"I can see clearly
now!"
An awakening to
cosmic awareness
Prayer and medi-
tation develop
healing

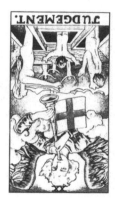

Judgement R
At a crossroads
Fears holding
you back
Frustrating delays
Inadequate
health care

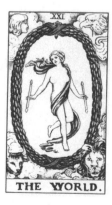

The World
Successful
culmination
Your new lifestyle
is ready!
Freedom to do as
you desire

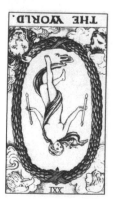

The World R
More work needed
to achieve goal
Life—and vitality—
is what you
make it!
You're almost there!

Tarot's Minor Arcana

Swords are Tarot's everyday suit of action in health; Wands, the suit of enterprise; Cups, the suit of emotions; and Pentacles, the suit of resources.

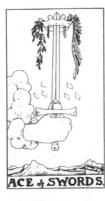

Ace of Swords
A new situation
or a new child
A new way of
communicating
Power: a sword
cuts two ways

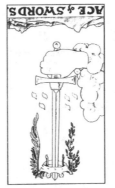

Ace of Swords R
The need to be
cautious and
vigilant
Beware of aggres-
sion or force
Listen before
acting

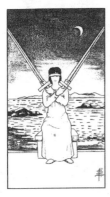

2 of Swords
Disconnected
from emotions
Indecision or
stalemate
Need to concen-
trate and focus

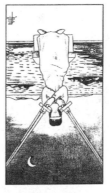

2 of Swords R
Remember to con-
nect to intuition
Use caution to
maintain balance
Freedom to make
decisions

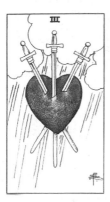

3 of Swords
Heartbreak and
sorrow
Pain, loss, and
grief
Learning about
loss and sadness

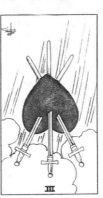

3 of Swords R
Passing sadness
Dissatisfaction,
but all is not lost
A different result
than what was
expected

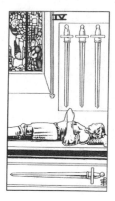

4 of Swords
R & R required!
Need for retreat
and meditation
Inner work being
done

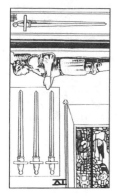

4 of Swords R
Ready for renewed
action
Ready to fight for
own rights
Opportunity to
change existing
condition

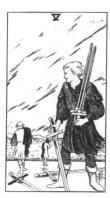

5 of Swords
Stormy weather
Someone taking
unfair advantage
Destructive
behavior, loss

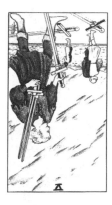

5 of Swords R
Feeling too weak
to fight
Gossip, sneaky
behavior
After conflict, the
truth is revealed

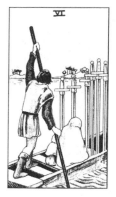

6 of Swords
Healing after
sorrow
Acceptance of
better things to
come
Leaving sorrows
and regrets
behind

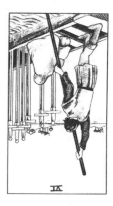

6 of Swords R
Stuck in a difficult
situation
Better to wait
and see
Delays, learn
to be patient

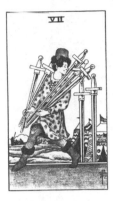

7 of Swords
Someone's being
sneaky
A need for the
truth to come out
Contradictions
and duality

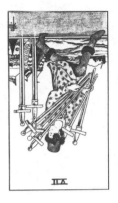

7 of Swords R
Wise counsel will
return
What was hidden
will be revealed
Freedom to
move on

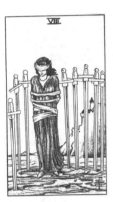

8 of Swords
Self-bound to
fears
Abuse of mental
power
Are you hurting
yourself the
most?

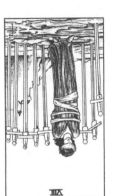

8 of Swords R
Letting go of fear
Facing one's own
restrictions
Hope returns,
movement is
freed

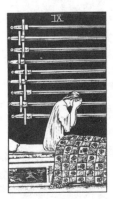

9 of Swords
Grief, sadness,
and sleeplessness
Learning to deal
with loss and
regret
Emotional
depression

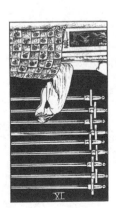

9 of Swords R
The nightmare is
over
Negative energy is
dissipating now
Worry falls away,
sleep returns

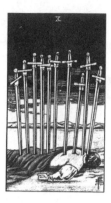

10 of Swords
End of a karmic
pattern
End of a difficult
cycle of treatment
Deep sense of
loss or separation

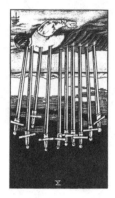

10 of Swords R
Releasing of a
karmic debt
Prepared to move
ahead
Health improve-
ment

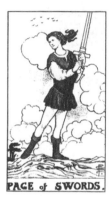

Page of Swords
Courage when
needed most
Using common-
sense approach
Pay attention to
details

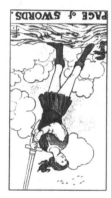

Page of Swords R
Overly emotional
communication
Need to speak mind
Importance of truth

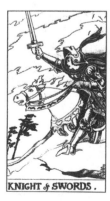

Knight of Swords
Sudden change of
direction
Direct honesty;
sometimes too
direct
Awakening to
truth

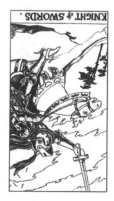

Knight of Swords R
Out of control!
Arguments and dis-
ruptive behavior
Lack of emotional
insight or stamina

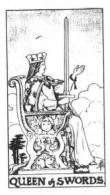

Queen of Swords
Ability to get to
the heart of the
matter
Joy of debate
Honesty and
forthrightness

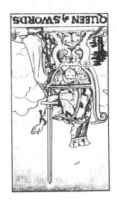

Queen of Swords R
Overly critical
person
Anxiety and mis-
communication
Judgmental or con-
tentious behavior

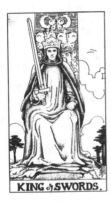

King of Swords
Logical analysis
Ability to probe
beneath surface
Rational counsel

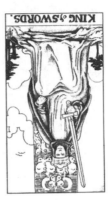

King of Swords R
Preconceptions
without basis
Stubbornness,
mental exhaustion
Selfishness, aloof-
ness

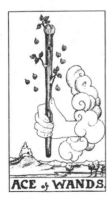

Ace of Wands
A fresh start
The first step
toward creating
your passion
A new relationship
or a new baby

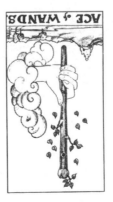

Ace of Wands R
Overenthusiasm gets
in your way
Delays or frustration
Need to regroup and
start again

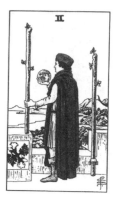

2 of Wands
Waiting for results
A good perspective
A positive attitude

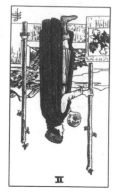

2 of Wands R
*Lack of follow-
through*
*Delays because of
others*
Rethink your plan

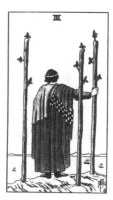

3 of Wands
*Cooperation and
partnership*
*Good results
forthcoming*
Help from others

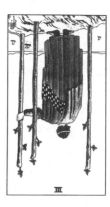

3 of Wands R
Wasted energy
*Inadequate
resources*
No one in the lead

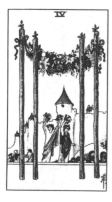

4 of Wands
*Family celebration
or ceremony*
*Contentment for
self and caregiver*
*A dream come
true*

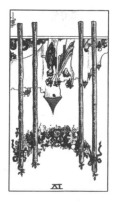

4 of Wands R
*Appreciating life's
little joys*
Thankfulness
*Enjoyment of small
pleasures*

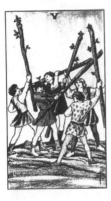

5 of Wands
Getting up on the
wrong side of the
bed
Disagreement
and crossed pur-
poses
Aggression and
misplaced energy

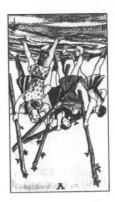

5 of Wands R
Problem-solving
and harmony
Negotiation and
constructive talks
Compromise and
conciliation

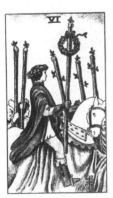

6 of Wands
Family reunion,
good news comes
home
A happy journey
with loved ones
Company is
coming

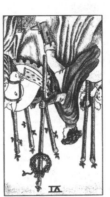

6 of Wands R
Stressful conditions
Need to ride out
the storm
Meditate on peace
of body/mind/spirit

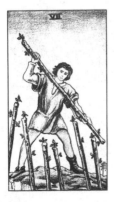

7 of Wands
Inner strength
and stamina
A good offense is
the best defense
Need to face
fears and turn
them around

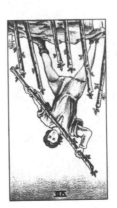

7 of Wands R
The storm is
passing
A sense of personal
empowerment
Progress toward
goals

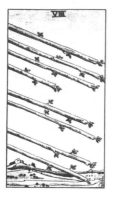

8 of Wands
Wands of good
health arrive!
Happiness and
progress
Goals within
reach, shared
passion

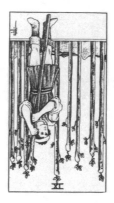

8 of Wands R
Disagreement and
discontent
Jealousy or anger
Reorganize toward
your goal

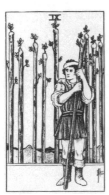

9 of Wands
Safeguarding
your health
Prepared to pro-
tect family, han-
dle adversity
Wisdom from
experience

9 of Wands R
Vulnerable and tired
Desire to be left
alone
Anxiety and poor
health

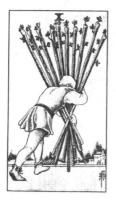

10 of Wands
Helping too
many others
at once
Stressful condi-
tions at home
Overwhelming
physical and
mental obliga-
tions

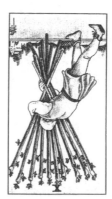

10 of Wands R
The burden is lifted
Learning to delegate
Taking the right
approach to respon-
sibility

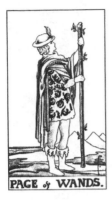

Page of Wands
A message of good news, encouragement
A child or a new child, a nurturing companion
Enthusiasm for life

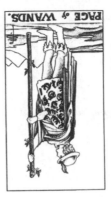

Page of Wands R
Disappointing news
Delay in receiving expected information
Preoccupied, unable to see the bright side

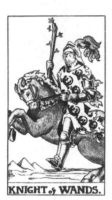

Knight of Wands
Enthusiasm and renewed energy
A new adventure
A generous loved one

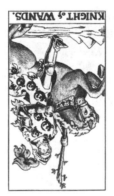

Knight of Wands R
Postponed journey
Disorganization and chaos
An unstable person

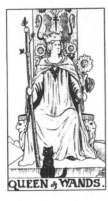

Queen of Wands
In command of domestic life
Someone who encourages others' self-sufficiency
Feminine ambition

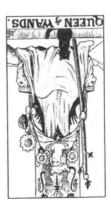

Queen of Wands R
Discomfort on the home front
Immature or domineering behavior
Confusion and obstinacy

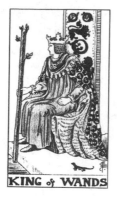

King of Wands
Someone willing
to lend a helping
hand
A good person
to have around
in a crisis
A passionate
mentor or proud
parent

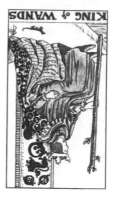

King of Wands R
Lack of confidence
and focus
Feeling grumpy
and detached
Pessimism or
doubt

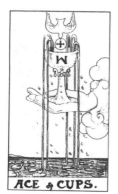

Ace of Cups
New beginnings
Opening of the
heart, joy
Fertility and con-
ception

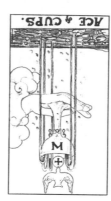

Ace of Cups R
Insecurity
Inability to con-
nect with others
Too much focus
on self

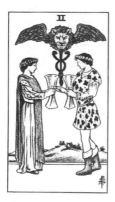

2 of Cups
Mutual emotional
understanding
Desire to build
alliance
Developing bal-
anced friendship

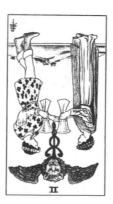

2 of Cups R
Misunderstanding
with a loved one
Negative emotions
Lack of balance in
relationship

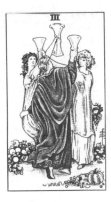

3 of Cups
Celebrating life,
vitality, abun-
dance
Happiness all
around
Great things
coming

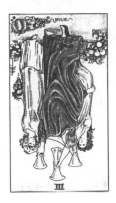

3 of Cups R
Disagreements,
unhappiness held
inside
Overindulgence,
petty emotions
Need for self-
control

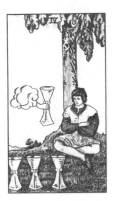

4 of Cups
Emotional detach-
ment, isolation
Need for inner,
spiritual work
Don't take health
for granted

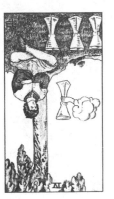

4 of Cups R
Ready to recon-
nect with others
Emotionally
ready for per-
sonal growth
Ability to visual-
ize and create
healthy you

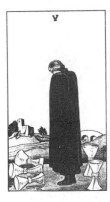

5 of Cups
Grief over loss
of vitality
Need to release
emotions, okay
to cry
Need to recog-
nize loss, heal

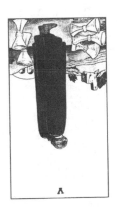

5 of Cups R
Return of posi-
tive energy and
hope
Letting go of
negativity
Knowledge
gained through
sorrow

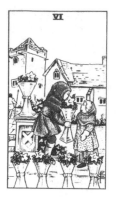

6 of Cups
Nostalgia for
family, past vital-
ity, health
An ally from the
past returns
Sharing good
memories

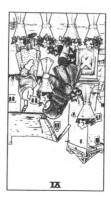

6 of Cups R
Hurtful past situ-
ation has current
echoes
Emotional need
to seek out the
past
Wishing for the
past instead of
the present

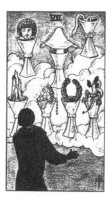

7 of Cups
Too many
choices!
Paying attention
to what is
beneath
Indecisiveness

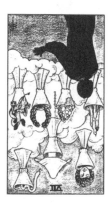

7 of Cups R
A treatment plan
has been made
Clarity among
choices
You finally took
action!

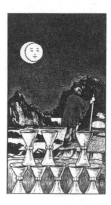

8 of Cups
Surrender to a
higher calling
Leaving the
material
Setting out on a
spiritual quest

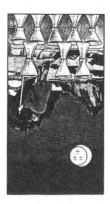

8 of Cups R
New alliance pos-
sible
Time to follow
your bliss
Taking pleasure
in life's good
things

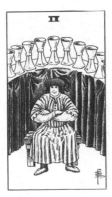

9 of Cups
Happy days are
here!
Your wish will
come true
Renewed vitality

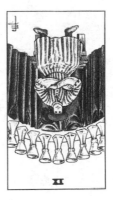

9 of Cups R
Expecting too
much
Wishes postponed
A need to develop
patience

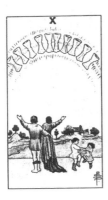

10 of Cups
The best support
network
Happily ever after!
Joy and happiness
in abundance

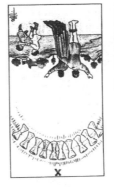

10 of Cups R
Not yet; another
piece to work on
Fear of ultimate
commitment
Troubled family
life

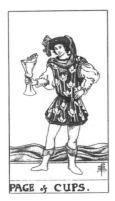

Page of Cups
Kindness and
compassion
Someone who
cares
Positive, joyful
energy, offer of
happiness

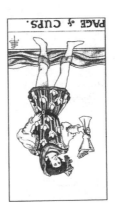

Page of Cups R
Someone is feeling
self-pity
Immature view;
melodramatic
Someone who is
oversensitive

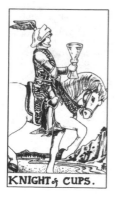

*Knight of Cups
Movement
toward a goal
New mentor or
guide is coming
Action toward
developing health*

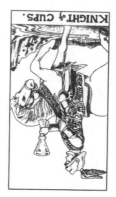

*Knight of Cups R
Vacillating
emotions
Emotionally
unable to give
Living in the past*

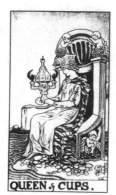

*Queen of Cups
Nurturing, car-
ing, person
A focus on sensi-
tivity
Someone with
great concern for
others*

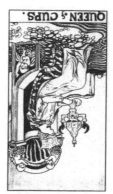

*Queen of Cups R
Emotionally exag-
gerates feelings
A worrier; an over-
active imagination
Tendency toward
secrecy or self-
deception*

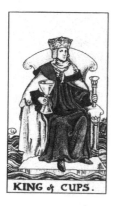

*King of Cups
Devoted, caring
person
Someone who
understands
others
A desire to help
others*

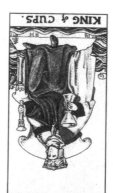

*King of Cups R
Recent emotional
loss
Emotional
detachment, hid-
den feelings
Potential for
manipulation of
feelings*

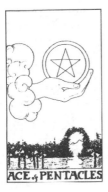

Ace of Pentacles
Focus on good
home environ-
ment
Good common
sense
Happiness of
solid foundation

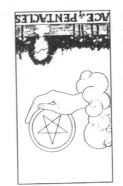

Ace of Pentacles R
Frustration and
delays
Need to hold tight
to what you have
Need to reassess
priorities

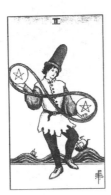

2 of Pentacles
Juggling more
than one thing
Confidence
despite stress
Balance is essen-
tial

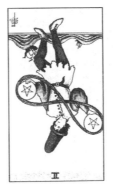

2 of Pentacles R
A hard time deciding
something
Need to simplify; let
something go
Need for caution

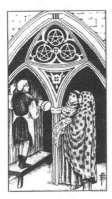

3 of Pentacles
A time to learn
new things
Approval for
work and talent
An award or
honor

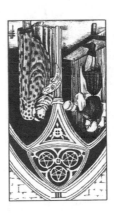

3 of Pentacles R
The reality
doesn't look like
the plan
Lack of passion
Sloppy workman-
ship

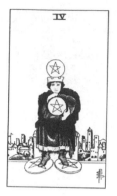

4 of Pentacles
Holding tight to
what you have
Conservative
about money
Careful about
insurance and
health issues

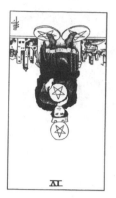

4 of Pentacles R
Spending more
than you have
Need to get or
address insurance
issues
Generosity; too
generous

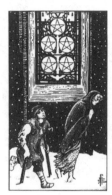

5 of Pentacles
A deep sense of
personal loss
Feelings of sep-
aration
Depleted re-
sources, turning
back on help

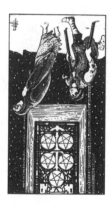

5 of Pentacles R
Renewed hope,
acceptance after
grieving
Negative cycle ends
Can now reap what
was sown

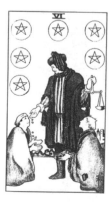

6 of Pentacles
Extra help is
offered
Sharing with
others
Financial reward;
a new job

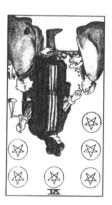

6 of Pentacles R
Be cautious of
what others offer
More giving than
taking
Unfair, unethical
behavior

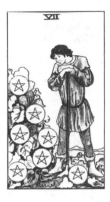

7 of Pentacles
Reaping the
rewards of hard
work
Payment for your
skill
Financial inde-
pendence

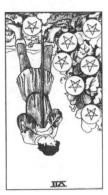

7 of Pentacles R
Poor speculation
Problems with
land or real estate
A need for caution
when speculating

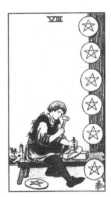

8 of Pentacles
Social approval
Development of
greater skill
Recognition for
job well done

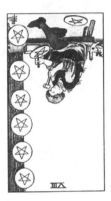

8 of Pentacles R
Delayed production
Lack of balance
in personal life
Someone is burning
out

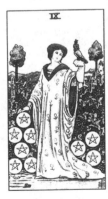

9 of Pentacles
The comforts
of home
Self-sufficiency
and independence
Prosperity to
share

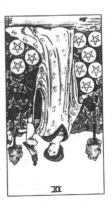

9 of Pentacles R
Financial insecurity
Anxiety at home
Uncertainty about
future

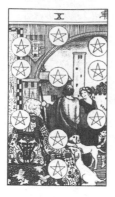

10 of Pentacles
*The height of
familial security
Multigenerational
security
A stable and
secure maturity*

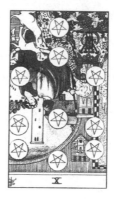

10 of Pentacles R
*Family feud!
Family wealth
at risk
Be cautious with
investments,
insurance*

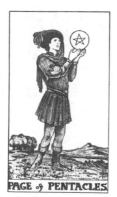

Page of Pentacles
*An eager learner
A message of
happiness
Good news;
good results*

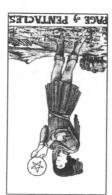

Page of Pentacles R
*A selfish or
demanding child
or person
Delays, differing
values
Prejudice or
rebellion*

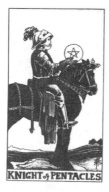

Knight of Pentacles
*Slow and steady
wins the race
Development of
prosperous future
Wise counsel and
good stewardship*

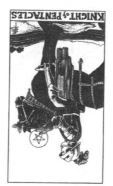

Knight of Pentacles R
*Discontent with pres-
ent work
Absent father figure
Irresponsibility,
slowed progress*

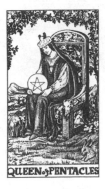

*Queen of Pentacles
Abundance, pro-
ductivity
The Earth Mother
personified
Always something
cooking on the
stove*

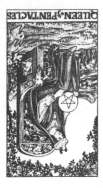

*Queen of Pentacles R
Financial insecurity
A lack of confidence,
needy, dependent
Losses in the home*

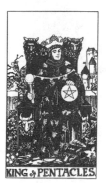

*King of Pentacles
A good parent
figure
Assured prosperity
Someone who will
share the wealth*

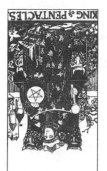

*King of Pentacles R
Laziness or lack of
motivation
Ill-equipped for
financial success
Disorganization,
discontent about
resources*

About the Authors

Arlene Tognetti grew up in a home where religion and spiritual ideas came together. Her mother, a traditional Catholic, and her father, a more Edgar Cayce–type individual, helped her to understand that there's more to this world than what's obvious. Arlene began studying the Tarot and Astrology in the 1970s and started her own practice in 1980. She began teaching the Tarot at the University of Washington in the Experimental College in 1982, and currently teaches the Tarot at Pierce College in Tacoma. Arlene's focus is on enlightening her students and clients: "I want everyone to learn what Tarot, Astrology, and Psychic Intuition are all about and how these Intuitive Arts can help them grow and look at the choices and alternatives in their lives." Arlene is expert author, with Lisa Lenard, of *The Complete Idiot's Guide to Tarot, Second Edition.* Arlene lives in the Seattle area. Her website is www.mellinetti.com.

Carolyn Flynn is a newspaper journalist and fiction writer with more than 20 years' experience. She is the editor of *SAGE Magazine,* a women's magazine that appears in the *Albuquerque Journal.* She lives in Corrales, New Mexico, where she spends most of her waking hours chasing her boy/girl twins. Her website is www.carolynflynn.com.

Amaranth Illuminare is a leading book producer, developing New Age and holistic wellness books for mainstream readers. Amaranth's goal: Touch readers' lives. In addition to *The Intuitive Arts* series, Amaranth has developed many books, including *Empowering Your Life with Joy* by Gary McClain, Ph.D., and Eve Adamson; *Releasing the Goddess Within* by Gail Feldman, Ph.D., and Katherine A. Gleason; and *Menu for Life: African Americans Get Healthy, Eat Well, Lose Weight, and Live Beautifully* by Otelio Randall, M.D., and Donna Randall. Amaranth's founder and creative director, Lee Ann Chearney, is the author of *Visits: Caring for an Aging Parent* and editor of *The Quotable Angel.*

The Intuitive Arts series

Use Astrology, Tarot, and Psychic Intuition to See Your Future

Discover how you can combine the Intuitive Arts to find answers to questions of daily living, use tools to help you see and make changes in your future, claim your brightest destiny, and fulfill your essential nature.

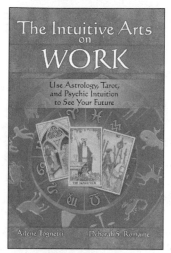

1-59257-108-5

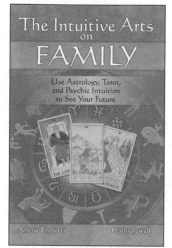

ISBN: 1-59257-110-7

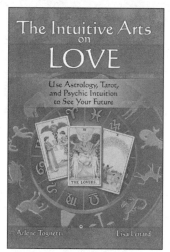

ISBN: 1-59257-106-9

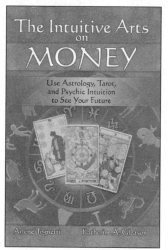

ISBN: 1-59257-107-7

ALPHA

A member of Penguin Group (USA) Inc.